T0296422

FAST FACTS ABOUT NURSING AND THE LAW

Paula DiMeo Grant, JD, BSN, MA, RN, is a nurse attorney admitted to practice law in the District of Columbia and currently is in private practice. Her experience includes litigation and mediation. From 1991 to 2011, she served as a mediator for the Superior Court of the District of Columbia, primarily mediating medical malpractice and personal injury cases. From 1998 to 2004, she served as of counsel to the law firm of Ross & Hardies and its successor McGuire Woods LLP. Ms. Grant, a registered nurse, received her BSN from Boston College and an MA in nursing education from New York University. She has developed legal nurse consulting programs and has lectured on nursing and the law, and published on these subjects. She is a member of Sigma Theta Tau International and is past president of the American Association of Nurse Attorneys Foundation. She is coeditor with Diana C. Ballard of *Law for Nurse Leaders: A Comprehensive Reference* (Springer Publishing Company, 2011).

Diana C. Ballard, JD, MBA, RN, is an experienced health care executive, health care attorney, and business owner. She has served in hospital executive management as chief nursing officer, vice president, and chief compliance officer. She is the owner of Ballard Consulting, offering services in business and program development, health care and health systems management, and customer service training. She was of counsel to the law firm of Susman, Duffy & Segaloff, PC, of New Haven, Connecticut, for 15 years, practicing in all aspects of health law. She has held adjunct faculty appointments at the University of Connecticut, Adelphi University, Yale University School of Nursing, University of New Haven, and University of Phoenix. She has taught and published extensively in health care and health law subjects. She has wide experience as a public spokesperson, keynote speaker, seminar leader, and broadcast media guest, including appearances on a weekly televised health series. She is the cocreator of CarePower®, a self-improvement approach to developing excellence in customer service. A Pace University Law School–educated attorney and registered professional nurse, Ms. Ballard holds a BS degree in psychology and an MBA. She is coeditor with Paula DiMeo Grant of *Law for Nurse Leaders: A Comprehensive Reference* (Springer Publishing Company, 2011).

FAST FACTS ABOUT NURSING AND THE LAW

Law for Nurses in a Nutshell

Paula DiMeo Grant, JD, BSN, MA, RN
Diana C. Ballard, JD, MBA, RN

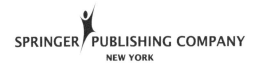

SPRINGER PUBLISHING COMPANY
NEW YORK

Springer Publishing Company, LLC
11 West 42nd Street
New York, NY 10036
www.springerpub.com

Acquisitions Editor: Allan Graubard
Composition: S4Carlisle Publishing Services

ISBN: 978-0-8261-1045-9
e-book ISBN: 978-0-8261-1046-6

13 14 15 / 5 4 3 2 1

The author and the publisher of this Work have made every effort to use sources believed to be reliable to provide information that is accurate and compatible with the standards generally accepted at the time of publication. The author and publisher shall not be liable for any special, consequential, or exemplary damages resulting, in whole or in part, from the readers' use of, or reliance on, the information contained in this book. The publisher has no responsibility for the persistence or accuracy of URLs for external or third-party Internet websites referred to in this publication and does not guarantee that any content on such websites is, or will remain, accurate or appropriate.

Library of Congress Cataloging-in-Publication Data
Grant, Paula DiMeo, author.
Fast facts about nursing and the law : law for nurses in a nutshell / Paula DiMeo Grant, Diana C. Ballard.
     p. ; cm.
Nursing and the law
Includes bibliographical references and index.
ISBN 978-0-8261-1045-9 — ISBN 0-8261-1045-2 — ISBN 978-0-8261-1046-6 (e-book)
I. Ballard, Diana C. (Diana Christine), 1945- author. II. Title. III. Title: Nursing and the law.
[DNLM: 1. Legislation, Nursing—United States—Handbooks.   2. Jurisprudence—United States—Handbooks. WY 49]
610.73—dc23   2012049528

Printed in the United States of America by Gasch Printing.

This book is dedicated to nurses—the heart of health care.

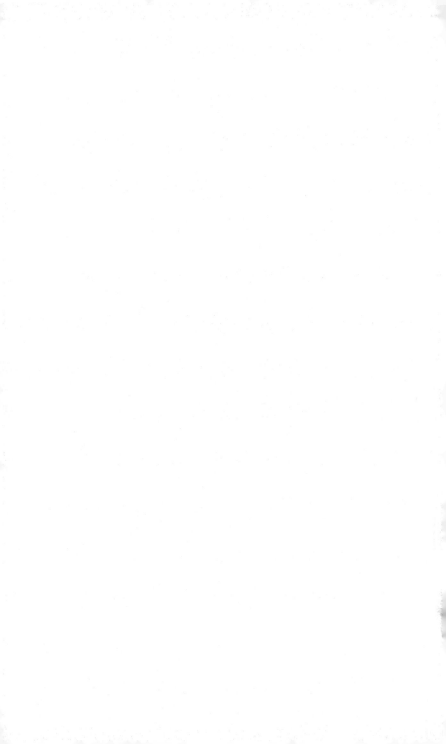

Contents

Part IV: Informed Consent and Patient Rights
Diana C. Ballard

Part V: Employment Law
Paula DiMeo Grant

Part VI: Organization and Business Law: Topics for Nurses
Diana C. Ballard

Part VII: Disasters and Public Health Emergencies
Diana C. Ballard

Part VIII: Resolving Disputes
Paula DiMeo Grant

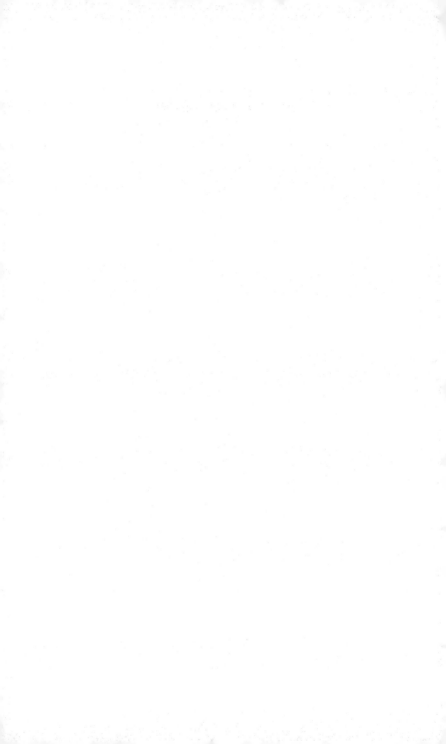

Preface

Nurses continue to hold a position of central importance in the world of health care, and this role will increase in the future. As we know, nurses are challenged every day by the latest clinical advances, new technology, and cutting-edge information based on science and research, to name a few areas.

In this ever-changing environment, this singular vital constant—nurses—must be able to practice their profession with knowledge and skill. In the practice of their profession, nurses are expected to make rapid decisions on critical issues. We understand that. We also understand that many decisions that the nurse is called upon to make have legal implications and therefore it is crucial that the decision be the best it can be.

This is why we wrote this book. This Fast Facts legal reference is intended to provide high-quality legal information *in a nutshell!* It is written for the nurse who is busy, who wants a ready reference, and who wants to obtain quality guidance in decision making as quickly as possible.

This reference covers many of the timely topics included in our earlier comprehensive text, *Law for Nurse Leaders: A Comprehensive Reference*. Recognizing that nurses will use that reference for more in-depth research, we created this book in response to the need for a quick and ready legal reference that will provide "on the spot" information.

The nurse will find valuable legal information on sources of law, Nurse Practice Acts, and the disciplinary process; nursing malpractice and negligence; documentation; informed consent and patient rights; employment; corporations, risk management, and compliance; disasters and public health emergencies; and dispute resolution.

Of course, we caution that the information provided in this book does not constitute legal advice and is not a substitute for competent legal representation. Only retained counsel, with full knowledge of any specific situation, can provide such representation and specific legal advice. However, in this book we have taken complex topics and presented them in straightforward, understandable language that you will find practical, useful, valuable, and indispensable.

As nurse attorneys, we are committed to providing you with the most relevant and useful information possible. We are confident you will find that we have accomplished that in this book.

Paula DiMeo Grant, JD, BSN, MA, RN
Diana C. Ballard, JD, MBA, RN

Acknowledgments

We are grateful to the many people who helped to make this book a reality.

We thank Springer Publishing Company for its constant and steadfast support and for its ongoing commitment to bring nurses the best possible resources. Allan Graubard, former Executive Editor at Springer, has been a genuine friend and gifted resource to us. We continue to benefit from all he has taught us. We also acknowledge the assistance and support of Assistant Editor Chris Teja for his invaluable and expert assistance in the production of this book. We are also grateful to Rose Mary Piscitelli, Senior Editor, and her team, who so capably led us to the finish line.

We are deeply grateful to the contributors of our earlier book, *Law for Nurse Leaders: A Comprehensive Reference.* Their outstanding contributions in the development of that first book were instrumental in the creation of this book. Their work is cited throughout this book with deep gratitude.

As always, we are able to count on the support of our friends and family, whose support and encouragement were given as enthusiastically in the writing of this book as they were with our first book. To our husbands, who have continued to be unwaveringly patient and supportive—to Paula's husband, Dr. James Grant, and to Diana's husband, John Capone—we express our heartfelt gratitude. Ms. Grant recognizes with love and gratitude her late parents, Samuel and Emilie DiMeo, and is forever grateful to them for inspiring her to be her best.

We, the authors, recognize each other with a level of respect and friendship that has not only made our achievements possible, but has made them a satisfying and fulfilling experience.

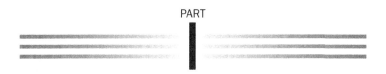

Overview of Nursing and the Law

Primary Sources of Law

Paula DiMeo Grant

The delivery of health care has become increasingly complex and requires nurses to have knowledge of the law as it relates to nursing practice and the care they deliver to patients. Part I: Overview of Nursing and the Law consists of three chapters and will focus on the primary sources of law, Nurse Practice Acts, the role and function of the Boards of Nursing, and the nursing disciplinary process. Case examples will illustrate salient points. Chapter 1 will address the four primary sources of law.

In this chapter, you will learn to:

1. Describe the four primary sources of law
2. Identify the source of law responsible for Nurse Practice Acts

FOUR PRIMARY SOURCES OF LAW

The four primary sources of the law consist of the following:

1. Constitutional Law
2. Common Law
3. Statutory Law
4. Administrative Law

Constitutional Law

The Constitution is the basic framework of our government, and parallel systems exist on both state and federal levels. Constitutional law is the interpretation and application of the principles as set forth in the Constitution. The United States Constitution guarantees basic rights to all U.S. born or naturalized citizens. The first 10 amendments of the U.S. Constitution are known as the Bill of Rights. The jurisprudence system ensures that these basic rights will not be infringed upon without due process of the law. The due process clause of the 14th Amendment of the U.S. Constitution states in part:

> No state shall make or enforce any law which shall abridge the privileges or immunities of the citizens of the United States; nor shall any state deprive any person of the life, liberty or property, without due process of the law; nor deny to any person within its jurisdiction equal protection of the laws.

Common Law

Common law is the body of law that is distinguished from law that is enacted by legislatures. It is a body of law that is derived from usage or custom, or from judgments or decrees of the courts. It is based upon the principle of precedent or *stare decisis*, which is Latin for "to abide by or adhere to" (*Black's Law Dictionary*, 1979). Common law originated in England and was later adopted by this country, and is often referred to as judge-made law or case law.

Statutory Law

Statutory law is law passed by the legislative branch of the state or U.S. government. It is a declaration that prohibits or demands certain actions to be taken or specific requirements to be met. Nurse Practice Acts are examples of statutory laws enacted by state legislatures.

Administrative Law

Administrative law is the area of law that is created by state and federal agencies or governing bodies. These agencies or governing bodies have rulemaking and adjudicatory powers. They promulgate rules and regulations and enforce administrative orders from matters adjudicated before an administrative law judge. The Boards of Nursing fall into this category.

=====*FAST FACTS in a NUTSHELL*

Common law originated in England and was later adopted in this country, and is often referred to as judge-made law or case law.

=====*FAST FACTS in a NUTSHELL*

State statutory law is primarily responsible for education, licensing, and regulation of nursing practice.

SUMMARY

The four primary sources of law as described in this chapter form the basic foundation for addressing the legal issues in nursing. As a result of the interrelatedness of law and nursing, and the changing landscape of the health care delivery system, it is important for nurses to have a basic knowledge of the law. The next two chapters of this book will focus on Nurse Practice Acts as well as the function of Boards of Nursing.

2

Nurse Practice Acts

Paula DiMeo Grant

Nurse Practice Acts (NPAs) are statutory laws enacted by state legislatures. Over the years, they have been amended to broaden the scope of nursing practice. The purpose of these acts is to assure the public that nurses meet certain educational and licensing requirements in order to safely practice nursing. NPAs define the scope of nursing practice and they also provide for the formation of a Board of Nursing to regulate and monitor practice. Broad powers are given to Boards of Nursing in carrying out their responsibilities. This chapter will discuss the purpose of NPAs, the nurse licensure compact, and the role of the Boards of Nursing.

In this chapter, you will learn to:

1. Explain the purpose of Nurse Practice Acts
2. Define the Nurse Licensure Compact
3. Describe the role of State Boards of Nursing

PROVISIONS OF NURSE PRACTICE ACTS

In 1903, North Carolina was the first state to enact the Nurse Practice Act (NPA), and other states followed. The practice of nursing is regulated by the states through their legislative authority. It is the power of the state to protect the health, safety, and general welfare of its citizens. This is also known as the states' police power; it is reserved for the states by the U.S. Constitution.

A typical NPA contains the following provisions:

1. Licensure requirements
2. Definition of the practice of nursing, including scope of practice
3. Authority for the formation of the Board of Nursing
4. Responsibilities of the Board of Nursing
5. Grounds for disciplinary actions, which may include license revocation or other lesser sanctions

The definition of professional nursing practice is important primarily for two reasons: (1) It delineates the areas of professional nursing, and (2) it protects the nurse from the charge of the unlicensed practice of medicine, as it did in the case of *Sermchief v. Gonzales* (1983), which is illustrated below (Grant, 2011, pp. 22–24).

CASE EXAMPLE

Sermchief v. Gonzales, 660 S.W. 2d 683 (Mo. Banc 1983)

Issue: Whether or not the nurse practitioners were practicing the unauthorized practice of medicine.

In the *Sermchief* case, nurses and physicians brought a petition for a declaratory judgment (which asks the court to establish the rights of parties or express an opinion of the court) and an injunction (which is a court order to stop a person from performing a specific act under certain circumstances) that the practices of nurses were authorized by the NPA and did not constitute the unauthorized practice of medicine. The petition further requested that the Medical Board be enjoined from taking any steps, either civil or criminal, to enforce the unauthorized practice of medicine against these parties.

The facts of the case are mainly undisputed. Appellant Nurses Solari and Burgess are RNs with postgraduate training in obstetrics and gynecology licensed to practice in Missouri. They are employed by an agency that provides medical services to the general public in the fields of family planning, obstetrics, and gynecology. The appellant physicians are also employed by the same agency and licensed to practice medicine (the healing arts) pursuant to Missouri statutes. They joined this action because they were charged with aiding and abetting the unauthorized practice of medicine by the nurses.

The respondents, meaning the parties answering the complaint, are the members and executive secretary of the Missouri State Board of Registration for the Healing Arts (Medical Board) and are charged with the responsibility of enforcing, implementing, and administering the rules and regulations of the Medical Board.

The services provided by the nurses and complained of by the board included, but are not limited to, history taking, breast and pelvic examinations, Papanicolaou (Pap) smears, gonorrhea cultures, blood serology, information about birth control, and the dispensing of certain medications.

The nurses were following written standing orders and protocols that were signed by the appellant physicians and specifically written for the nurses Solari and Burgess. No act by the nurses is alleged to have caused injury or harm to any person.

LOWER COURT'S DECISION: The lower court denied the petition, and the case was appealed to the Missouri Supreme

Court, which reversed the decision and held that services routinely provided by nurses and complained of by the Board of Registration for the Healing Arts fell within the legislative standard of "professional nursing."

APPELLATE COURT'S DECISION: The Supreme Court, in reversing the decision and remanding the case, that is, sending it back to the Lower Court, stated:

The Nursing Practice Act of 1975 substantially revised the law affecting the nursing profession by redefining the term "professional nursing" to expand the scope of authorized nursing practices permitting nurses to assume responsibilities heretofore not considered to be within the field so long as those responsibilities were consistent with the nurses' specialized education, judgment, and skill.

In 1975, the Missouri legislature made a substantive change in the NPA, which had a positive outcome for this case. The court went on to say, "[the] professional nursing standard provided in the amended statute did not constitute the unlawful practice of medicine, where nurses' diagnoses were within the limits of nurses' respective knowledge and nurses referred patients to physicians upon reaching limits of their knowledge" (p. 683).

The court also said, "the hallmark of the professional is knowing the limits of one's professional knowledge" (p. 690). In this matter, the nurses made the proper referrals to the physicians in accordance with the written protocols. In reversing the Lower Court's decision, this case is significant in that it represents the broadening of the scope of nursing practice that was authorized by the legislature and recognized by the Appellate Court.

The *Sermchief* case is an example of the application of the law and the expansion of the NPA, as it was applied to the facts of the case in reaching a decision by the court.

Nurse Licensure Compact

In order to facilitate nursing practice across state lines, the Nurse Licensure Compact (NLC) was formed. This compact allows for registered nurses (RNs) and licensed practical nurses (LPNs) to have a multistate license in their primary state of residency and to practice, physically or electronically, across state lines in other states that recognize the NLC, unless the nurses' practice is restricted. Table 2.1 illustrates the states that participate in the compact. Advanced practice registered nurses (APRNs) are not included in this compact. Nurses should familiarize themselves with the NPA of each state in which they are licensed to practice nursing. In the event that disciplinary action is taken in one state, the nurse may also be subject to discipline in another compact state. For additional information on NLC, visit www.ncsbn .org/nlc (Grant, 2011).

Scope of Nursing Practice

The scope of nursing practice is defined by the Nurse Practice Act (NPA); it refers to the legally permissible boundaries of practice, depending on the educational background of the nurse. The scope of nursing practice is extremely complex as a result of various nursing specialties and the advanced practice of nursing. Nurses are assuming greater responsibility and accountability as the demands for the delivery of nursing care are increasing.

The scope of practice has been dealt with on different levels, including legislative amendments to the NPA expanding nursing practice, as well as courts applying the law to cases involving practice issues, as previously illustrated by the *Sermchief* case. In addition, violations of NPAs are routinely addressed by Boards of Nursing when complaints against nurses regarding practice are filed.

TABLE 2.1   Nurse Licensure Compact States

1. Arizona
2. Arkansas
3. Colorado
4. Delaware
5. Idaho
6. Iowa
7. Kentucky
8. Maine
9. Maryland
10. Mississippi
11. Missouri
12. Nebraska
13. New Hampshire
14. New Mexico
15. North Carolina
16. North Dakota
17. Rhode Island
18. South Carolina
19. South Dakota
20. Tennessee
21. Texas
22. Utah
23. Virginia
24. Wisconsin

Source: NCSBN (2010).

FAST FACTS in a NUTSHELL

The practice of nursing is regulated by the states through its legislative authority by the enactment of Nurse Practice Acts. It is the power of the state to protect the health, safety, and general welfare of its citizens.

Boards of Nursing

Boards of Nursing consist of nurses and lay individuals appointed by the governors of each state to serve specified terms of office. The purpose of the board is to safeguard the public from the unlawful and unsafe practice of nursing. This is accomplished by the regulation of nursing education and licensure. The board is responsible for approving the educational programs for RNs, LPNs, and licensed assistive personnel. In addition, the board has the authority to issue or deny a license to practice nursing. The board monitors nursing practice by evaluating all complaints or allegations of violations of the NPA or other rules that may place patients in harm's way. The nursing disciplinary process will be discussed in the next chapter. Boards of Nursing have broad powers to fulfill their duties and responsibilities. Each board has an executive director to carry out the day-to-day operations.

FAST FACTS in a NUTSHELL

The purpose of the Board of Nursing is to safeguard the public from the unlawful and unsafe practice of nursing. Boards have broad powers to regulate nursing practice.

SUMMARY

Nurse Practice Acts define the scope of nursing practice and contain the legal parameters of practice. Each state has enacted its own Nurse Practice Act. The Nurse Licensure Compact was formed to facilitate nursing practice across state lines, with states having the authority to issue multistate licenses. Certain criteria must be met, and not all states participate in the compact. It is strongly advised that nurses be familiar with the Nurse Practice Act in each state where they are licensed to practice nursing. Boards of Nursing have broad powers to regulate and monitor the practice of nursing. Members of the board are appointed by state governors to serve specified terms of office.

3

Nursing Disciplinary Process

Paula DiMeo Grant

This chapter will describe the nursing disciplinary process and the role of the Board of Nursing in that process. There will be a discussion of the steps taken when a complaint alleging violations of nursing practice or any other conduct subject to review is brought before the board against the nurse. There will also be a comparison of discipline versus alternative programs for impaired nurses and reporting mechanisms.

In this chapter, you will learn to:

1. Define the role of the Board of Nursing
2. Identify the stages in the nursing disciplinary process
3. Explain what constitutes unprofessional conduct
4. Describe alternative programs for impaired nurses

BOARDS OF NURSING

The nursing disciplinary process is one of the major functions of the Boards of Nursing. The boards are state governing bodies authorized to conduct investigations and hearings, request the production of evidence, and subpoena witnesses. In the discharge of its duties, the board may also deny a nurse an application for licensure or relicensure. Boards may also sanction nurses for violations of the Nurse Practice Act (NPA) or other rules and regulations by the revocation or suspension of a nursing license. Nurses may also be placed on probation, or the board may institute conditions placed upon the licensee following a hearing or settlement. Due process of the law affords the nurse notice and a hearing based upon the charges brought by the board against the nurse, and an opportunity to refute those charges. It is important for the nurse to consult with a competent attorney should he or she receive notification from the Board of Nursing regarding any allegation of violations of the NPA or other rules and regulations.

═══════════════════════════════════*FAST FACTS in a NUTSHELL*

The nursing disciplinary process is one of the major functions of the Boards of Nursing.

Commencement of a Disciplinary Action

A nursing disciplinary action usually begins with a complaint filed against the nurse before the Board of Nursing, alleging specific violation(s) of nursing practice or the inability of the nurse to safely practice because of an impairment. In most states, impaired nurses are offered an alternative to disciplinary action, which will be discussed later in this chapter. As a general rule, the violations of nursing practice can fall into the broad category of "unprofessional conduct." The definition of unprofessional conduct can be found in the NPAs or laws governing nursing practice. Nurses should be familiar with what constitutes unprofessional conduct in the state where they practice. The definition varies from state to state.

Unprofessional Conduct

Unprofessional conduct may include any of the following activities:

1. Fraudulent or deceptive procurement or use of a license.
2. Advertising that is intended to or has the tendency to deceive.
3. Failing to comply with provisions of state or federal statutes or rules governing practice of the profession.
4. Failing to comply with an order from the board, or violation of any term or condition of a license given by the board.
5. Practicing the profession when medically or psychologically unfit to do so.
6. Delegating professional responsibilities to a person whom the licensed professional knows or has reason to know is not qualified by training, experience, education, or licensing credentials to perform them.
7. Willfully making or filing false reports or records in the practice of the profession and willfully impeding or obstructing the proper making of or filing reports or records or willfully failing to file the proper reports or records.
8. Failing to make available promptly to a person using professional health care services, that person's representative, succeeding health care professionals or institutions, upon written request and direction of the person using

professional health care services, copies of that person's records in the possession or under the control of the licensed practitioner.

9. Failing to retain client records for a period of 7 years, unless laws specific to the profession allow for a shorter retention period. When other laws or agency rules require retention for a longer period of time, the longer retention period shall apply.

10. Conviction of a crime related to the practice of the profession or conviction of a felony, whether or not related to the practice of a profession.

11. Failing to report to the office a conviction of any felony or any offense related to the practice of the profession in a Vermont district court, a Vermont superior court, a federal court, or a court outside Vermont within 30 days.

12. Exercising undue influence on or taking improper advantage of a person using professional services or promoting the sale of services or goods in a manner that exploits a person for the financial gain of the practitioner or third party.

13. Performing treatments or providing services that the licensee is not qualified to perform or that are beyond the scope of the licensee's education, training, capabilities, experience, or scope of practice.

14. Failing to report to the office within 30 days a change of name or address.

15. Failing to exercise independent professional judgment in the performance of licensed activities when that judgment is necessary to avoid action repugnant to the obligations of the profession.

    (b) Failing to practice competently by reason of any cause on a single occasion or on multiple occasions may constitute unprofessional conduct, whether actual injury to a client, patient or customer has occurred. Failure to practice competently includes:

(1) Performance of unsafe or unacceptable patient or client care, or

(2) Failure to conform to the essential standards of acceptable and prevailing practice.

(c) The burden of proof in a disciplinary action shall be on the state to show by a preponderance of evidence that the person engaged in unprofessional conduct. (3 V.S.A. Section 129(a) 1–15, (b) 1, 2, (c)).

As one can see from this example of unprofessional conduct in the state of Vermont, the behaviors listed cover a wide range of misconduct, from failure to notify an address change to failure to practice competently, or any felony charge.

FAST FACTS in a NUTSHELL

A nursing disciplinary action usually begins with a complaint filed against the nurse before the Board of Nursing alleging violations of nursing practice or the inability to safely practice nursing as a result of an impairment.

Stages in the Disciplinary Process

Stage One: Complaint Reviewed

The Board of Nursing staff, upon receiving a complaint against a nurse for violations of nursing practice, will evaluate the allegations to determine whether or not they are sufficient to require an investigation by the board or a referral to an alternate program.

Stage Two: Decision Made to Investigate or Refer

Stage two involves the initial decision made by the board after review of the complaint.

This decision may include one of the following actions:

1. The case is NOT OPENED by the board because the information submitted is insufficient to warrant an investigation of the allegations in the complaint.
2. The case is OPENED for investigation and assigned to an investigator or investigative team. The nurse is notified in writing of allegations made in the complaint against him or her.
3. The case may be REFERRED to an alternative program, depending upon the charges and the state where the charges are brought. Alternative programs address the impaired nurse.

Stage 3: Investigation

The Board of Nursing opens a case and reviews the allegations made against the nurse in the complaint. The investigative team may include a staff investigator, a board member, and a prosecuting attorney. The investigator will request copies of written documentation and any relevant records pertaining to the complaint. Witnesses may be interviewed and the nurse may be requested to submit information in the form of answering questions in writing. The investigator will present evidence submitted for review. If the evidence submitted is not adequate to support a finding of violations of the NPA or of other rules and regulations, a recommendation not to pursue formal charges will be made and the case or complaint will be closed.

Stage 4: Formal Charges Against Nurse by Board

Following the investigative phase, if the evidence is sufficient, formal charges will be filed against the nurse by the Board of

Nursing pursuant to the statutory requirements of the state where the charges are filed. The prosecuting attorney will draft the charges in the form of allegations that are made in the complaint and supported by evidence obtained by the investigative team. The nurse receives the formal charges, and the process is no longer confidential. Upon advice of counsel, the nurse will answer the charges. The answer generally takes one of three forms:

1. An admission of the allegation(s)
2. An admission with an explanation
3. A denial of the allegation(s)

═══════════════════════════*FAST FACTS in a NUTSHELL*

If a nurse receives notification of an action brought before the Board of Nursing, consultation with competent counsel is recommended.

Stage 5: Settlement Agreement or Hearing

The allegations and the answers to those allegations by the nurse will form the basis for a hearing before an Administrative Law Judge. The nurse will be afforded due process in accordance with the law. If the nurse so chooses, he or she can forgo a hearing and enter into a Settlement Agreement or Consent Agreement negotiated by the nurse and his or her attorney and the Board of Nursing. A settlement agreement allows some control over the process. However, entering into an agreement and forgoing a hearing should not be taken lightly and should be done only after careful consideration because all appeal rights are lost. The Settlement Agreement will contain specific terms and conditions depending on the nature of charges; it may have sanctions and may require probation and educational courses. Disciplinary actions are reportable to the national data banks.

In the alternative, the nurse may choose to have a formal hearing before an Administrative Law Judge, who has the authority to hear cases and render decisions based upon the evidence presented. The government or prosecuting attorney has the burden to prove all the allegations against the nurse by a preponderance of evidence or by clear and convincing evidence in order to find the nurse has violated the NPA or other rules and regulations pertaining to practice. The hearings are conducted in accordance with the state's Administrative Procedure Act and local rules of the court. The nurse will have an opportunity to submit relevant evidence and present witnesses to refute the allegations in the complaint. Once a decision is made, following a formal hearing, either party may appeal to a court of law (Grant, 2011).

Alternative Disciplinary Programs

Alternative disciplinary programs have been established by State Boards of Nursing to address the problem of nurses impaired by substance abuse disorders and mental illnesses. The substance abuse disorders refer to a wide range of conditions from abuse to dependency or addiction to alcohol or drugs. The American Nurses Association (ANA), as reported by the National State Boards of Nursing (NSBN), has estimated that 6% to 8% of nurses are impaired to the extent that it affects professional performance. Nurses entering into alternative disciplinary programs must meet certain criteria as established by the particular State Board of Nursing (NSBN, 2012). Alternative disciplinary programs offer nurses an opportunity for rehabilitation, which is confidential in nature and generally is not reportable to data banks.

Alternative Program Model

As a result of the passage of the Nurses Rehabilitation Act of 2000, the District of Columbia established a Committee On Impaired Nurses (COIN). Its purpose is to provide an alternative to disciplinary actions taken by the Board of Nursing for nurses who are impaired as a result of dependency on drugs or alcohol, or suffering from mental illness.

The committee is charged with monitoring the recovery of nurses to ensure the safe practice of nursing. Unlike disciplinary action, information regarding the nurse's participation in the COIN Program is confidential and all records are destroyed 2 years after the nurse completes the program.

COIN Program Admission

The parameters of admission to the program include:

1. Self referrals or reports by the impaired nurse
2. Formal complaints
3. Referrals by the Board of Nursing

A nurse enters the program on a voluntary basis provided that he or she does not have a record of arrests or convictions for the diversion of controlled substances for distribution or sale. Further, the nurse does not have a history of causing patient injuries.

Participation Agreement

When the nurse accepts participation in the program, he or she is required to sign a Participation Agreement that contains certain terms and conditions, which may include the following:

- Working conditions (e.g., hours, practice areas)
- Progress reports from treatment program
- Limitations on the administration of controlled substances
- Random drug and alcohol screening
- Reports from supervisor
- Self-reports

COIN participation is confidential and not reportable to data banks (The District of Columbia Board of Nursing Committee on Impaired Nurses [DCBON], 2012).

═══════════════════════════*FAST FACTS in a NUTSHELL*

Alternative Disciplinary Programs have been established to address the problem of impaired nurses.

SUMMARY

Boards of Nursing have broad regulatory powers to license and monitor the performance of nursing practice in their respective states. Nurses should be familiar with what is deemed unprofessional conduct or misconduct in the states in which they are licensed to practice nursing. In the event that a nurse is notified of a complaint regarding practice issues brought before the Board of Nursing, it is wise for him or her to consult with a competent attorney as soon as possible. Nurses have a right to due process of law when allegations of violations of nursing practice are made against them.

Nursing Boards have addressed substance abuse issues by offering nurses participation in alternative programs instead of taking disciplinary action. These programs are confidential in nature and, unlike disciplinary actions taken by the board, are generally not reportable to data banks. Nurses should remain vigilant and knowledgeable in the area of disciplinary actions taken by Boards of Nursing.

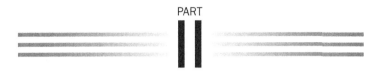

Nursing Malpractice/Negligence

4

Negligence/Malpractice

Paula DiMeo Grant

Nurses have made great strides over the years on their journey to professionalism, and have had increased responsibilities and accountability. As a result, they have been subject to malpractice actions when standards of nursing care have been breached. Part II will focus on Nursing Malpractice/Negligence and the nurse as an expert witness. Most malpractice cases require expert testimony to prove malpractice. This chapter will cover the definition of negligence/malpractice and the elements necessary to prove the nurse's negligence in a court of law. Defenses to the action will also be discussed. Standards of nursing care will be reviewed, and a list of areas of nursing malpractice will be provided. Case examples will be utilized to demonstrate important points. The terms negligence and malpractice will be used interchangeably.

In this chapter, you will learn to:

1. Define malpractice/negligence
2. Identify the elements needed to prove malpractice actions
3. Discuss the standards of nursing care
4. Identify defenses to malpractice actions
5. Describe common areas of nursing negligence/malpractice

A FOCUS ON NEGLIGENCE/MALPRACTICE

Negligence/Malpractice Defined

Negligence is defined as the failure to exercise the standard of care that a reasonably prudent person would exercise in the same or similar circumstances (*Black's Law Dictionary*, 2004). When an allegation of negligence is made, the conduct is compared with the conduct of what a reasonably prudent person would have done in the same or similar circumstances (Karno, 2011). When a nurse–patient relationship is established, a negligent act can occur by the nurse's commission of a duty to act or by the nurse's omission of a duty to act. Not all omissions or commissions of duty by the nurse rise to the level of nursing malpractice. For malpractice to occur, the law requires that certain elements must be proven.

═══════════════════════════*FAST FACTS in a NUTSHELL*

Negligence is defined as the failure to exercise the standard of care that a reasonably prudent person would exercise in the same or similar circumstances (*Black's Law Dictionary*, 2004).

Four Elements Necessary to Prove Negligence/ Malpractice

In order to prove that the nurse was negligent, the plaintiff (injured party bringing the action) must prove, by a preponderance of evidence, the elements of a negligence action. The four elements are:

1. A duty owed
2. Breach of duty owed

3. Causation (proximate)

4. Damages

Duty

The first element to be proven in a negligence matter is that there was "a duty owed" by the nurse to the patient. A nurse–patient relationship must be established to meet this element of negligence. Typically, this relationship begins when the nurse is assigned to care for patients in a hospital or other setting.

Breach of Duty

The second element to be proven in a negligence action is that the nurse breached the duty owed to the patient by failing to provide the proper standard of care for his or her nursing actions. The plaintiff must prove that the standard of care fell below the acceptable standard at the time that the breach occurred. In most instances, the breach of the standard of care is established by expert testimony.

Proximate Cause

The third element necessary to be proven in a negligence action is that of proximate cause. *Proximate cause* means that the nurse's failure to provide the appropriate standard of care by an omission or commission of an act was the "cause in fact" of the injury. For example, if the nurse failed to give a patient a dose of Coumadin and the patient did not suffer consequences even though the standard of care was breached, the omission does not constitute negligence/malpractice, because there was no proximate cause of injury, the third necessary element.

Damages

The last or fourth element that must be proven by the plaintiff is that the injury caused the plaintiff to sustain damages. Compensable damages include both economic and noneconomic damages. Economic damages are awarded to the prevailing plaintiff for loss of income, medical expenses, and other out-of-pocket expenses. Noneconomic damages are awarded to the plaintiff for pain and suffering, emotional injuries, and permanent and partial disabilities as a result of the injuries sustained. All four elements must be proven, by a preponderance of the evidence, for a finding of malpractice.

══════════════════════FAST FACTS in a NUTSHELL

Four elements are needed to prove negligence/malpractice: (1) duty, (2) breach of duty, (3) proximate cause, and (4) damages.

Standards of Care

The law requires that the nurse's conduct conform to the applicable standard of care as set forth by the profession. "The standard of care is a legal concept and has been judicially defined by the courts as the exercise of the same degree of knowledge, skill and ability as an ordinarily careful professional would exercise under similar circumstances (Karno, 2011, p. 253; *Seavers v. Methodist Medical Center of Oak Ridge*, 1999).

It is important to note that the standard of care is continually changing as scientific and technological advances take place. (The nurse's conduct will be judged by the standard of care in effect at the time the allegations of malpractice occurred.) Therefore, nurses need to stay current with the standards of care by reviewing the Nurse Practice Act, the American Nurses Association (ANA) Code of Ethics, agency and employer policies and procedures, nursing specialty standards of practice, nursing textbooks and journals, and any other sources of the standards of nursing practice. Continuing nursing education programs, nursing conferences, and in-service education programs provide the nurse with current knowledge regarding nursing practice and the standards of nursing care.

==*FAST FACTS in a NUTSHELL*

In a malpractice action, the nurse's conduct will be judged by the standard of care in effect at the time the incident occurred.

Joint and Several Liability

Liability means that one is legally obligated or responsible; in the context of medical malpractice, it pertains to the one(s) found to have caused the injuries or damages suffered by the plaintiff. Joint or several liability is when two or more parties are responsible together or individually (*Black's Law Dictionary*, 2004). For example, in a malpractice case, the plaintiff can bring a suit against one or more physicians and one or more hospitals. The amount of damages remains the same regardless of the number of wrongdoers. A plaintiff can recover the damages from both wrongdoers or from either wrongdoer. The plaintiff does not receive double compensation (Karno, 2011).

Negligence/Malpractice Defenses

The defenses in a negligence/malpractice action include the following:

1. Statute of limitations
2. Contributory or comparative negligence
3. Charitable or sovereign immunity
4. Good Samaritan acts
5. Failure to prove malpractice

Statute of Limitations

If a claim of malpractice is not filed timely by the plaintiff, it may be time-barred, and the case may be dismissed by the court. States have enacted statutory law with time limits in which to bring a lawsuit; the time period varies from state to state. Those laws are called the statute of limitations. There are, however, exceptions to the usual statute of limitations regarding negligence or malpractice actions which include minors and incompetent individuals, allowing for a longer period of time to bring a claim.

Contributory or Comparative Negligence

In some jurisdictions, contributory negligence by the plaintiff will bar complete recovery for injuries sustained. This defense is based upon the fact that the conduct of the plaintiff caused the injury or harm suffered, and therefore the defendant should not be held liable. Comparative negligence, on the other hand, will reduce the amount of recovery in proportion to the negligence of the plaintiff. For example, if the plaintiff was 20% at fault and was awarded damages amounting to $60,000, the award would be reduced by $12,000, or 20%. The plaintiff would receive $48,000 instead of the award of $60,000. This reduction occurs by operation of law.

A threshold limit called "modified comparative negligence" has been adopted in some jurisdictions. In those jurisdictions, the plaintiff will be barred from recovery of any damages if he or she is more than 50% negligent (Karno, 2011).

Charitable or Sovereign Immunity

The doctrine of charitable and sovereign immunity exempts an individual or entity from liability under certain conditions. Historically, nonprofit hospitals were protected from lawsuits under the doctrine of charitable immunity, and government health care delivery systems were protected under the sovereign immunity doctrine. While both immunity doctrines are being eroded, the statutory immunity provisions of the law do not prevent a lawsuit from being filed. Rather, the immunity provision provides a basis for dismissal by the judge. Moreover, immunity is not absolute where the alleged professional negligence is found to be willful, reckless, or of a gross nature (Karno, 2011).

Good Samaritan Acts

The Good Samaritan statutes enacted by the state legislatures, as the name implies, give protection from lawsuits when health care providers administer emergency care in emergent situations when there is no duty to act. Although the laws vary from state to state, immunity is granted from liability for negligent acts and is predicated on the fact that care is provided in good faith and without fear of lawsuits. Nurses should stay current with the Good Samaritan laws.

Failure to Prove Negligence

In order to prevail in a court of law, the plaintiff is required to prove all four elements of negligence: a duty, a breach of duty, proximate cause, and damages. If one or more of those elements is missing, the verdict will be for the defendant.

Areas of Nursing Malpractice

The following list represents some of the areas of nursing practice that have resulted in nursing malpractice actions:

1. Medication errors
2. Failure to follow policies, procedures, and treatment protocols
3. Failure to properly assess, observe, or monitor patients
4. Failure to document changes in a patient's condition

5. Untimely or no proper notification of a patient's deteriorating condition

6. Inappropriate delegation of duties

7. Improper documentation

8. Patient abandonment

9. Failure to maintain a safe environment for patients

10. Failure to follow prescribed orders

11. Failure to determine or document allergies

12. Failure to provide patients with adequate discharge instructions and teaching

CASE EXAMPLE

Medication Error

Harris County Hospital District v. Estrada (1993)

Summary of Facts: Carolina Gonzalez, a 73-year-old woman, received her routine care at the West End Medical Clinic. She presented to the clinic with complaints and symptoms of an infection. She was examined by Dr. John Bradberry, a Baylor College of Medicine resident physician. She was given a prescription for Bactrim, not withstanding her documented history of allergy to sulfa drugs. Mrs. Gonzalez suffered a severe allergic reaction and expired 16 days later.

Nursing Allegations

- Failure to review medical record documentation for history of allergies.
- Failure to maintain appropriate documentation of history.
- Failure to provide adequate discharge instructions regarding adverse reactions to medication.

COURT PROCEEDINGS: Before filing the lawsuit, the Gonzalez family settled with Bradberry and Baylor College of Medicine. The family subsequently sued the clinic for the nursing allegations. The plaintiff's nursing expert testified that it was the discharge nurse's independent duty to compare the prescription with the patient's medical record for contraindications, such as allergies, and to bring any inconsistencies to the attention of the physician. In addition, the nurse expert testified that the discharge nurse also has a duty to instruct the patient on the symptoms of an adverse reaction and what to do in the event of a reaction. The nurse expert further testified that the sole proximate cause of the inappropriate prescription and death was the negligent record-keeping by the clinic's nursing staff.

A second nurse expert testified that the clinic nursing staff had a duty to review the prescription with the plaintiff, provide discharge instructions, and advise the plaintiff to seek immediate medical attention in the event of a drug reaction. Evidence was presented showing that a drug reaction can be reversed if treated quickly.

The examining physician testified that he relied on the clinic's computer printout that showed Gonzalez had no allergies. The computer printout and patient record are given to a physician upon examination of a patient.

The computer sheet is a summary of the medical data contained in the patient record prepared by the medical records clerk. The nurse failed to review the patient record or verbally confirm any allergy history with the patient. The jury determined that the nurse's failure to meet the standard of care for documentation requirements and discharge instructions was a proximate cause of the allergic reaction and subsequent death.

COURT'S DECISION: The jury returned a guilty verdict against the nurse and awarded damages to the Gonzalez family.

This case illustrates the importance of the nurse's independent review of the patient's record. As this case demonstrates, there can be risk involved in depending on physicians, clerks, and computers for critical information such as patient allergies. This case also exemplifies the need for proper discharge instructions and patient teaching regarding drug interactions and the appropriate interventions (Karno, 2011).

Liability Insurance Coverage

Nurses should consider obtaining their own malpractice insurance coverage. Insurance considerations should be carefully explored. At the time of employment, the nurse needs to have a clear understanding of the type of liability coverage the employer is offering. Generally, employer insurance coverage will be effective only during the time of employment, and will not cover any incident outside the scope of employment. This is a good reason for nurses to carry their own individual liability insurance policy. Insurance policies contain many terms and conditions and should be fully understood by the nurse. Independent contractors and/or agency nurses should pay special attention to liability insurance coverage.

It is important to note that there are some liability insurance policies that also cover nursing disciplinary defense matters brought by Boards of Nursing.

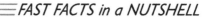

FAST FACTS in a NUTSHELL

Nurses need a clear understanding of their malpractice insurance coverage.

SUMMARY

Nurses have gained professional autonomy and recognition; with those gains have come increased accountability and responsibility. As a result, nurses continue to be named as defendants in medical malpractice actions. Nurses need to remain knowledgeable as to the current standards of nursing care in order to deliver optimal care to patients in all settings. Malpractice/negligence is based on an unintentional act (omission or commission) by the nurse in delivering patient care. When malpractice is alleged, the plaintiff is required to prove all four elements of negligence as discussed in this chapter. The ever-changing health care landscape continues to present challenges to nurses across all health care settings. It is imperative that nurses remain knowledgeable regarding any changes in the Nurse Practice Act or changes in policies and procedures in the delivery of nursing care.

5

Proving Malpractice: The Expert Nurse Witness

Paula DiMeo Grant

The expert nurse witness plays an important role both in and out of the courthouse. This chapter will focus on the role and purpose of the expert witness. Qualifications of the expert will be discussed as well as preparation, including case evaluation and testimony. A recent and important case example regarding nurses serving as expert witnesses will be reviewed. Most malpractice actions, with very few exceptions, require an expert witness to prove whether or not malpractice has occurred. The terms malpractice *and* negligence *will be used interchangeably.*

In this chapter, you will learn to:

1. Define the role of the expert nurse witness
2. Discuss the importance of the expert nurse witness in nursing malpractice actions
3. Identify resources for expert nurse preparation
4. Discuss advances made by nurses in serving as expert witnesses

EVOLUTION OF THE EXPERT NURSE WITNESS

In general, the evolution of the role of the expert nurse witness mirrors that of the nursing profession. Historically, nurses were not viewed as professionals and consequently were not considered to have the requisite qualifications to serve as expert witnesses. Nursing education, state laws, and court decisions have shaped the progress that nurses have made on their journey to professionalism (Grant, 1998). Depending upon the nature of the case, the minimum requirement to serve as an expert witness is a current license to practice professional nursing.

In the past, it was common for a physician to testify as to whether or not the standard of nursing care was breached. This approach was used in the wrongful death case of *Haney v. Alexander* (1984), when a North Carolina Appellate Court upheld a decision of a trial court in allowing a physician to testify that a nurse breached the standard of care by failing to adequately monitor the vital signs of the decedent as his condition worsened and ultimately led to his death.

A different approach, however, was taken in the *Sullivan v. Edward Hospital, et al.* (2004) case as illustrated below.

CASE EXAMPLE

Sullivan v. Edward Hospital et al. (IL. S. Ct., 2004)

Issue: Whether or not a board-certified internist was competent to testify as to the standard of care of a nurse in a malpractice action.

SUMMARY OF FACTS: The facts of this case reveal that a 74-year-old male was admitted to the hospital for a urinary tract infection. He had a history of suffering a stroke and was partially paralyzed. It was reported that although he could not speak, he was able to understand. During the evening shift, he attempted to get out of bed and became agitated. The evening nurse notified his treating physician and requested a Posey restraint. Instead, the physician ordered a sedative, which was administered. Although he was monitored, he fell out of bed, struck his head, and sustained a head injury as a result. (He expired in 1999 from an unrelated event.)

In 1998, this case was filed against the treating physician and the hospital. The complaint alleged that the hospital, through the nurse and the physician, failed to monitor, medicate, and restrain the plaintiff. Damages were sought for negligence. At trial, the plaintiff called a board-certified internist to testify as to the applicable standard of nursing care. The physician expert testified as to his extensive experience working with doctors and nurses in the area of patient fall protection.

His testimony included a deviation from the standards of nursing care in three areas: (1) the nurse failed to notify her supervisor that the patient was a fall risk, (2) the nurse's failure to provide an alternative to the Posey restraint, and (3) the nurse's failure to properly communicate the patient's condition to the physician (The American Association of Nurse Attorneys [TAANA], 2007).

LOWER COURT'S DECISION: The Trial Court entered a directed verdict for the hospital because the plaintiff's only medical expert was ruled incompetent to testify as to the standard of care for the nursing profession. A directed verdict is a ruling made by the trial judge that takes the case from the jury because the evidence will permit only one reasonable verdict (*Black's Law Dictionary,* 2010). There was a jury verdict in favor of the defendant physician.

APPELLATE COURT'S DECISION: The Appellate Court affirmed the decision as did the Supreme Court of Illinois. TAANA submitted an Amicus Brief (friend of the court) on behalf of the defendant, and the Supreme Court in its ruling cited the TAANA brief.

The profession of nursing has evolved into its own separate and distinct body of knowledge from the profession of medicine, as evidenced by the Sullivan case. Nurses have increasingly served as expert witnesses in courtrooms and as consultants to attorneys in health care–related matters. In some jurisdictions, physicians can testify as to whether or not the standard of nursing care was breached, although that practice is being eroded.

FAST FACTS in a NUTSHELL

Nurses have increasingly served as expert witnesses in and out of the courtroom.

ROLE OF THE EXPERT NURSE WITNESS

Expert testimony is required when the trier of fact (judge or jury) needs to make a decision that falls outside of their knowledge and understanding. In nursing malpractice litigation, the expert nurse witness is necessary to determine the standard of nursing care and whether that standard has been breached. The underlying question in every nursing malpractice action is whether or not the nurse's specific acts or omissions conformed with the standard of care at the time the incident occurred. The responsibilities of the expert witness may include the following tasks:

1. Analysis of medical records and/or medical reports
2. Review of applicable standards of care and nursing literature
3. Determination of whether or not the standard of care was breached
4. Identification of injuries caused by the breach
5. Submission of written opinion of findings
6. Testimony at a deposition
7. Testimony at trial

The hiring attorney and the expert witness will determine the scope of the expert's responsibilities and compensation. The expert nurse will first determine the parties involved and whether a conflict of interest exists. It is important to resolve those issues at the beginning.

===*FAST FACTS in a NUTSHELL*

Expert testimony is required when the trier of fact (judge or jury) needs to make a decision that falls outside their knowledge and understanding.

RESOURCES FOR EXPERT PREPARATION

The following is a list of some of the resources that the expert nurse witness may use in preparation:

1. Nurse Practice Act
2. ANA's Code of Ethics
3. ANA's Standards of Nursing Practice
4. Nursing Specialty Organizations Standards of Practice
5. Agencies' policies and procedures manuals
6. Occupational Safety and Health Administration (OSHA) rules and regulations
7. The Joint Commission standards and regulations
8. Licensing regulations
9. Textbooks, journals, and articles
10. Case decisions

An effective expert nurse witness is one who is thoroughly prepared and is knowledgeable about the standards of nursing practice as it applies to the case at hand. The witness will present his or her opinion in a confident and convincing manner. It is the duty of the witness to educate the trier of fact (judge or jury) regarding the health care–related issues. There will be an expert for the plaintiff (injured party) and also one for the defendant (nurse or physician or both).

If a malpractice lawsuit has already been filed, it is also important that the nurse review the trial documents submitted by all parties. The attorney will provide the pertinent documents for review by the expert witness. The expert may be required to give a deposition (testimony under oath) before trial; see chapter titled "Anatomy of a Trial" for additional information on depositions.

QUALIFICATIONS OF EXPERT WITNESSES AT TRIAL

If scientific, technical, or other specialized knowledge will assist the trier of fact to understand evidence or determine a fact in issue, a witness qualified as an expert by knowledge, skill, experience, training, or education may testify thereto in the form of an opinion or otherwise (F.R.E. 702, 2011). Most state courts have adopted the same qualifications as the federal rule.

It is the nurse's education, knowledge, experience, and skills that enable him or her to provide testimony in a court of law. The minimum requirement is a current license to practice professional nursing.

METHOD OF EXPERT QUALIFICATION

The hiring attorney will qualify the expert nurse witness by asking a series of questions on direct examination at trial. The following is a sample of the questions that may be asked:

1. Please state your name and address.
2. What is your educational background?
3. What professional licenses do you hold?
4. What certifications do you have?
5. What is your nursing experience?
6. Where are you employed?
7. What is your title?
8. Do you hold any leadership positions?
9. Have you published any nursing articles or books?
10. Have you received any nursing awards?

(Grant & Reardon, 2011)

FAST FACTS in a NUTSHELL

The judge determines whether the expert is qualified, and the jury determines the expert's credibility.

PRESENTATION OF TESTIMONY BY EXPERT

The above questions lay the foundation for the judge to accept or reject the nurse as an expert. After the nurse's acceptance as an expert, the attorney will ask the expert for his or her opinion and the basis for the opinion. The nurse should present his or her opinion in a confident and convincing manner to the jury. It is the jury that determines the credibility of the witness (Grant, 1998).

The nurse will, in all likelihood, be cross-examined by opposing counsel. The purpose of cross-examination is two-fold: (1) to elicit favorable testimony to enhance the position of the opposing side and (2) to discredit or impeach the expert witness. It is important for the nurse to answer only the questions asked.

The expert witness with a strong educational background, including certification in a specialized area of nursing practice, and with good communication skills will be one who is credible and persuasive before the judge or jury. Remember, thorough preparation remains the key. For additional information, see the chapter titled "The Anatomy of a Trial."

FAST FACTS in a NUTSHELL

In the past it was common for the physician to testify as to whether or not the standard of nursing care was breached; that practice is being eroded, as evidenced by recent case law. The trend is to have nurses testify instead.

SUMMARY

As rapid changes in health care continue, the need for expert nurse witnesses will become greater, both in and out of the courthouse. Nurses serving as experts provide an invaluable service to the profession. Their testimony impacts decisions made by judges and juries and has profound effects on the profession of nursing and on our system of jurisprudence. The decision to serve as an expert nurse witness rests solely with the nurse.

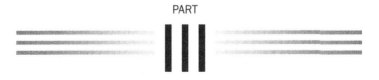
Documentation

6

Principles and Practices
of Documentation

Diana C. Ballard

Medical records are legal documents reflecting clinical practice. A patient's medical record needs to be a reliable record of all of the care provided to the patient. In the case of a legal proceeding in connection with the patient's care, the medical record will be examined to see if the care the patient received was provided according to the proper standard of care and in concert with applicable law and regulation. A well-documented record could also provide an effective defense for a health services provider who is alleged to have committed professional malpractice.

This chapter reviews the uses of the medical record, the contents of the medical record, and fundamental practices for creating and maintaining a proper medical record. Information on the basic practices applies whether working with manual or computerized systems, as it addresses proper practices with regard to creation of the medical record rather than the means used to create the record.

In this chapter, you will learn:

1. The purposes and uses of the medical record
2. The contents of the medical record
3. The fundamental characteristics of a well-maintained record

PURPOSE AND FUNCTION
OF THE MEDICAL RECORD

Laws governing medical records vary among states. Either through licensure laws or by other means, a record of all care and treatment provided to a patient in a medical setting must be kept. Law and regulation can emanate from both state and federal sources. Nurses should know the legal requirements with regard to medical records in their area of practice and in their jurisdiction.

In addition to being in compliance with law and regulation, records of patient care are maintained for other reasons. These reasons include:

- Communication and continuity of care among providers
- Clinical research purposes
- Performance improvement evaluation
- Regulatory compliance
- The creation of a permanent record of care provided to a patient
- Evidence that can be used in a legal or regulatory proceeding

CONTENTS OF THE MEDICAL RECORD

In all cases, the written record of patient care provides evidence of the care and services a patient received. The record should clearly show what services and care the patient received; when the services were received; what response or reaction the patient had to the services and treatment; who provided the service; what medications the patient received; and whether communication to other providers was carried out. In short, virtually everything that happens to a patient during a course of care and treatment should be evident from reading the medical record. This would be the case whether the record was handwritten, computerized, or some combination of both.

===============*FAST FACTS in a NUTSHELL*

Medical records must be complete and accurate. Everything that happens to a patient during care and treatment should be entered in the record.

KEY ASPECTS OF MEDICAL RECORD DOCUMENTATION

General Principles

Each page of the medical record must identify the patient by at least two identifiers, such as name, date of birth, or medical record number. Handwritten entries must be legible, unambiguous, and written in black or blue indelible ink. Every entry must have a complete date and time that permit an accurate reconstruction of the sequence of events. Every entry must be signed by the person making the entry. Nurses must sign entries using the last name as it appears on their nursing license, and the signature should indicate status such as RN or CRNA. With hand-generated records, avoid leaving empty spaces on the page, as this provides an opportunity for another person to alter the record, either intentionally or inadvertently (Brous, Boulay, & Burger, 2011).

Timing of Events

One of the most important characteristics of a well-documented medical record is that it specifies when care and treatment were given. For example, the record should specify the precise time a medication was given, when vital signs were actually obtained, when a physician was notified, or when an intervention actually occurred. The medical record should tell the complete story of the patient's care and treatment, and the story should be specific, accurate, and reliable.

Every entry into the medical record should indicate the complete date and time the note is being written, as well as the date and time of the event or observation being documented, and must be signed by the individual making the entry.

=== *FAST FACTS in a NUTSHELL*

One of the most important characteristics of a well-documented medical record is that it accurately and precisely specifies when care and treatment were given.

Sometimes it is necessary to make a so-called late entry, or to correct an entry that was made in error. Nurses must be diligent when making any proper change to the medical record, and must do so in compliance with the rules governing such actions in their facility or care setting.

Late entries must be identified as such. When charting the occurrence of an event or observation, or when adding information to a previously written entry, the note should clearly indicate that it is being written as an addendum or late entry. By so doing, there is a clear and accurate reconstruction of events, and the record is more likely to be viewed as credible, since the reason for the late entry has been explained.

Corrections to the medical record must be made in accordance with the organization's policy. Any procedure to correct a medical record entry must assure that the original entry remains readable. In general, an entry is corrected by drawing a single line through the incorrect entry so that the original entry that is under the cross-out line can still be read. The person making the new entry should sign above the line and add words such as "incorrect entry," or whatever words the organization's policy dictates. With regard to electronic records, corrections should be made according to the organization's policy. Of course, pencil entries, scribbles, correction fluid, erasures, and similar techniques should not be used in a medical record (Brous, Boulay, & Burger, 2011).

======================*FAST FACTS in a NUTSHELL*

Corrections to the medical record must be made in accordance with the organization's policy, which must assure that the original entry remains readable.

Specifically with regard to handwritten entries, if the notes continue from one page to another, they should be identified as continuation notes. At the end of the first page, the word "continued" should be added and signed by the person making the entry. The next page, where the note continues, should start with "continued from" with the date and time of the entry being completed, and of course, should also be signed. This method allows an accurate chronology and ensures that notes can be read in their entirety (Brous, Boulay, & Burger, 2011).

Records that do not provide an accurate and reliable record of the sequence of events leave questions about the specifics of care unanswered, and in a legal review this can be problematic. Records of lab tests and procedure records, direct testimony of witnesses, and testimony of experts are used to fill in gaps resulting from an incomplete record. However, the best and most direct and reliable record of events is that which is written into the medical record at or as close to the time of the event as possible.

Complete and Accurate Records

Medical records must be complete and accurate. Incomplete, missing, altered, or destroyed medical records give rise to noncompliance with regulatory standards, potential tampering of evidence, violation of an organization's policies, and departure from the proper standard of practice.

Medical records must accurately record events and reactions that are expected as well as those that are unexpected. They must also provide an accurate record of adverse events. In other words, all information critical to the complete record of the patient's care and treatment must be included in the record. Failure to document critical information regarding an adverse event can lead to the appearance of a cover-up. Further, falsifying a medical or business record is criminal activity and may also be considered professional misconduct by a nursing review board.

Use of Abbreviations

Any abbreviations, symbols, acronyms, or dose designations used in the record must be approved for use pursuant to the stated policy of the organization. If this procedure is followed, a provider who comes across an abbreviation that he or she does not recognize can look it up on the organization's approved list. This helps to ensure accuracy and promote safety for the patient (Brous, Boulay, & Burger, 2011).

Communication

An area of high risk and an issue that is critical is the reporting of changes in a patient's condition. Allegations such as a nurse's failure to monitor for changes, failure to recognize changes in condition, failure to report changes to the physician, and failure to intervene on behalf of the patient in a timely manner can only be adequately refuted when the relevant information is present in the medical record. Courts have held that nurses are responsible for communicating their findings to physicians and may be held liable for failing to do so (Brous, Boulay, & Burger, 2011).

Nursing documentation must clearly reflect that the patient is being monitored for foreseeable complications, recognizing them in a timely fashion and identifying concerns to the physician. Flow sheets are often used to record frequent assessment of a patient's condition, and properly filled out flow sheets can constitute a record of adequate assessment of the patient's condition (Brous, Boulay, & Burger, 2011).

When making an entry with regard to notification of a physician in such cases, the note should clearly identify which physician was advised of the findings and what time the notification was made. These elements should be made with specificity.

The nurse is required to pursue any concerns about the condition of the patient to final resolution. It is not enough to simply record in the chart that the physician was called. The nurse must ascertain that the physician has been notified. If the nurse encounters difficulty in fulfilling this responsibility, then he or she should pursue resolution using the problem-solving procedures available in his or her organization.

=*FAST FACTS in a NUTSHELL*

The nurse is required to pursue any concerns about the condition of the patient to final resolution. For example, it is not enough to say "physician's office notified." Rather, the nurse must ensure that actual notification of the physician has occurred.

SUMMARY

A patient's medical record must reliably, accurately, and completely record all of the care and services provided to the patient. The record must be in compliance with laws, regulations, and the organization's policies and procedures. A well-documented medical record can provide an effective defense for a provider who is alleged to have committed professional malpractice.

7

Electronic Health Records

Diana C. Ballard

Electronic health records (EHRs) are the wave of the future. Legislation at the federal level, namely the American Recovery and Reinvestment Act of 2009 (ARRA), the Patient Protection and Affordable Care Act of 2010 (ACA or Affordable Care Act), and the Health Information Technology for Economic and Clinical Health Act (HITECH), directs the Centers for Medicare and Medicaid Services (CMS) to offer incentives to providers for the adoption and meaningful use of EHR technology (Brous, Boulay, & Burger, 2011).

Among the many benefits attributed to the use of EHRs are enhanced speed and accuracy of documentation, improved communication across providers and disciplines, inclusion of error prevention mechanisms, avoidance of problems associated with illegibility, and provision of cross-communication with billing, performance evaluation, and management systems.

In this chapter, you will learn:

1. The key legislative initiatives associated with the transition to EHRs and their effect on the development of EHRs
2. The major challenges for nurse leaders associated with development, implementation, and use of computerized documentation systems
3. Key aspects of specialized documentation systems such as OASIS (Outcome and Assessment Information Set) and medication-dispensing systems

DEFINITION OF ELECTRONIC HEALTH RECORDS

An electronic health record (EHR) is the official health record for an individual when it exists in digital format. Like the paper version of the medical record, the EHR includes the record of the care and treatment provided to a patient. Based on the level of development in a facility, the medical record may be totally or partially in digital format. Bolstered by federal incentives to ultimately require medical records to be in digital format, EHRs are capable of being shared across different health care settings. In some cases this sharing can occur by way of network-connected enterprise-wide information systems and by other information networks or exchanges.

EHRs can include all elements of the medical record, such as progress notes, flow sheets, nursing and other disciplines' care plans, databases, teaching plans, baseline and ongoing assessments, evaluative statements, and anticipated outcomes. When fully developed, integrated, and well used, they may, among other things, increase speed of charting, increase accuracy and help to avoid error, produce management and patient classification reports, and project future patient care staffing needs.

BENEFITS OF EHRs

A feature of electronic recordkeeping that can enhance care and communication across disciplines is through the automatic population of fields. For example, vital signs recorded by the nurse can automatically be carried over to other disciplines and caregivers via the electronic record. Not only does this make important information immediately available to other disciplines that may need it, but it also avoids redundant entries and possible discrepant records (Brous, Boulay, & Burger, 2011).

Also of great importance, such issues as illegibility, erasures, and corrections are eliminated, as electronic records are automatically time- and date-stamped for each entry and the documentation records are legibly computer-generated (Brous, Boulay, & Burger, 2011).

The program can include prompts for mandatory data, and if the data are not entered, the computer can send an instant visual or audible notification. Care standards can be tailored for the specific patient population. If data entered are outside the range of standard expectations, alerts can appear that require the nurse to perform a range of different actions. Once a patient profile is created and entered into the system, it is available for review on subsequent admissions or episodes of care (Brous, Boulay, & Burger, 2011).

========================*FAST FACTS in a NUTSHELL*

The extent to which the benefits of EHRs are effective is dependent on the design, functionality, and use of the EHR system.

PRIVACY

The Health Insurance Portability and Accountability Act (HIPAA) of 1996 (P.L.104-191) Title II of HIPAA, known as the Administrative Simplification (AS) provisions, required the establishment of national standards for electronic health care transactions and national identifiers for providers, health insurance plans, and employers. One of the chief objectives of this law is to ensure privacy of health care records (Brous, Boulay, & Burger, 2011).

Computerized systems have a greater potential for harm due to unauthorized access or release of private information. This is due to the large amount of personal health data contained in such systems. Organizations must have systems in place to track usage and to detect unauthorized access or system breaches. Policies should include penalties for discovered instances of such occurrences. Organizations should also provide comprehensive privacy training so that all employees are informed as to the consequences of unauthorized conduct in connection with personal health information.

SECURITY

Privacy issues are addressed through use of a unique name and password. Where appropriate, the system can require a second signature, such as when associated with the use of controlled substances or high-risk medications. Of course, nurses and other system users should not disclose their name and unique password, as this might result in unauthorized entries attributed to the nurse or user whose password was revealed.

As with the use of any computer system, the nurse must take care to avoid unauthorized or fraudulent entries made under his or her name. For example, if the nurse who is logged in to the system walks away from the computer station, leaving the record open, another person can then access the patient record and make entries. The entered information, whether correct or not, is entered under the previous user's name. Thus, the record will no longer reflect the care provided to the patient as recorded by the practitioner who was actually logged on (Brous, Boulay, & Burger, 2011).

This is an avoidable situation. The safest practice is to log off from the computer terminal when moving away from it. If this is not done and the record is left open, it is vulnerable to alteration by another person. Organizations have strict procedures and rules with regard to system and user security, and nurses are advised to be diligent in complying with such procedures—for their own safety and that of the patient!

══════════════════════FAST FACTS in a NUTSHELL

It is important to be sure to log off from the computer terminal when moving away from it. If this is not done and the record is left open, it is vulnerable to alteration by another person.

ABBREVIATIONS, ALTERATIONS, AND ERROR CORRECTION

Software programs can be programmed to reject attempts to use unauthorized abbreviations. The system can be programmed to reject any abbreviation, acronym, or other shortcut that is not on the organization's approved list.

System design can also make it difficult to alter a record that has been automatically closed. For example, a record may remain open in the system during hospitalization but will close or "time out" within hours of discharge (Brous, Boulay, & Burger, 2011).

Facilities should have specific procedures and policies in place for error correction. Timely correction of errors is critical, as the system's timing-out feature may close a record before the correction can be made. An uncorrected error results in an inaccurate record and can be interpreted as an impropriety. In addition, the automatic date and time stamp, as well as the correction procedure employed, has the benefit of clearly documenting the fact of an error correction (Brous, Boulay, & Burger, 2011).

HEALTH SYSTEM REFORM AND EHRs

Moves toward EHRs have been shaped by various legislative initiatives. This was accomplished by the American Recovery and Reinvestment Act of 2009 (ARRA), the Patient Protection and Affordable Care Act of 2010 (ACA or Affordable Care Act), effective March 2010, and the Health Information Technology for Economic and Clinical Health Act (HITECH), with the final rule released on July 13, 2010, by the Centers for Medicare and Medicaid Services (CMS). Not all provisions of these acts are immediately in effect or enforceable. However, it is important to familiarize yourself with current and future requirements (Brous, Boulay, & Burger, 2011).

ARRA and ACA are new laws with great significance and influence on systems of documentation. They authorize CMS to offer incentives to providers for the adoption and meaningful use of certified EHR technology through the provisions of HITECH. Under these rules, certain eligible professionals, hospitals, and critical access hospitals could qualify for monetary incentives for efforts to adopt, implement, or upgrade certified EHR technology for meaningful use, based on specific objectives and measures for each care setting (Brous, Boulay, & Burger, 2011).

The following offers a general summary with regard to the incentives:

- Physicians, nurses, and nurse midwifes who are not hospital based and whose patient volume is at least 30% attributable to Medicare would be eligible for up to 85% of their net allowable technology costs, subject to specific annual limits.
- Medicaid incentives will be available only to non-hospital-based clinicians, encompassing dentists, certified nurse midwives, and physician assistants practicing in rural health clinics.
- Medicaid incentives range up to $65,000 over a 5-year period.
- Acute care hospitals whose Medicaid patient volume is 10% or more of their total volume, and children's hospitals with any Medicaid volume are also eligible.
- Medicaid has not mentioned any penalties for lack of adoption of EHRs.
- After obtaining start-up funds, providers who will prove meaningful use can be eligible to receive payments up to $10,000 annually for an additional 4 years. (Brous, Boulay, & Burger, 2011)

The Congressional Budget Office (CBO) estimates that approximately 90% of doctors and 70% of hospitals will be using EHRs within the next decade as a result of ARRA.

The HITECH portion of the laws can affect nurses who work in clinics, independent nursing practices, medical offices, and home care, where referrals for care that is medically necessary must originate. The incentive program will provide payments for efforts to adopt, implement, or upgrade certified EHR technology, but they must also demonstrate "meaningful use" of this technology according to the specific objectives. Simply purchasing a certified system is not enough (Brous, Boulay, & Burger, 2011).

Further, the rules will develop standards for all certified EHR systems and require that all systems speak the same language. This will allow the efficient exchange of information among providers and between providers and CMS. A central goal of this concept is the improvement of health care and prevention of Medicare and Medicaid fraud and abuse. As these laws are extensive and complex, capable counsel should be retained to assist with their full interpretation and understanding (Brous, Boulay, & Burger, 2011).

COMPUTERIZED MEDICAL RECORDS IN HOME HEALTH

In 2000, in the Budget Reconciliation Act of 1997, CMS instituted a home care documentation system that was intended, but not required, to be computerized. This was the now familiar home health documentation system Outcome and Assessment Information Set (OASIS). OASIS is the documentation system required under laws that govern home care for Medicare and Medicaid beneficiaries (42 U.S.C. 1395, et seq., 42 C.F.R. 409 et seq.). It is now usually computerized but can be filled out manually in whole or in part. The system utilizes fill-in forms for certain standardized demographic and general information, social and health history, living arrangements, review of systems, and medications and equipment management assessments. In all, there are seven dozen categories of information that can be used to evaluate each home care client (Brous, Boulay, & Burger, 2011).

OASIS is the form used during home health visits and is complemented by an interdisciplinary plan of care and progress notes, both of which, while in standardized format, necessitate a narrative approach. The new EHR rules will need to be analyzed to determine what effect, if any, they may have with regard to the current OASIS system (Brous, Boulay, & Burger, 2011).

AUTOMATED MEDICATION DISPENSING SYSTEMS

Automated medication dispensing systems are technology that is used to improve safety, provide access, and improve unit operations while providing tracking and record-keeping capability in connection with medication administration. Several manufacturers of these systems have been in use throughout the United States since the 1980s. The systems automatically link the facility pharmacy to the point of care. This provides the patient care unit with enhanced record-keeping capability. It is a passive collection of data, which means that the data are collected and recorded by the operation of the system itself. This provides medication administration data from which administrators and staff can have access to information about usage and trends. The system may also provide bar coding technology for the nurse, and electronic patient profiling that aids in dispensing medications by confirming the positive identification of patients with the correct medication, dose, time, and route of administration. Use of bar coding and medication administration systems can reduce or minimize the possibility for medication administration errors (Brous, Boulay, & Burger, 2011).

A key feature of these systems for nurses is the legal protection afforded by a system that is designed to provide accurate documentation. When medication is removed from the unit, the system creates an automatic computerized record in real time of the information about the medication and when it was pulled from the drawer and dispensed to the patient (Brous, Boulay, & Burger, 2011).

═══════════════════════════*FAST FACTS in a NUTSHELL*

Key to all electronic, automated systems is the assurance that they are well designed, do what they are supposed to do reliably and accurately, and do not fail.

SUMMARY

EHRs are the wave of the future, bolstered by federal incentives and legislation. They can enhance patient care and communication across disciplines and health care providers. When fully developed, properly designed, and effectively used, they can increase the speed of charting, increase accuracy, assist in prevention of error, and produce valuable reports. Computerized systems have a greater potential for harm from unauthorized access to, or release of, private information than do manual systems. Therefore, organizations should have systems in place to train users and monitor system use.

8

Keys to Reducing Liability

Diana C. Ballard

*This chapter discusses the establishment of legal stan-
dards for documentation systems in general. The system selected must meet basic legal requirements, and the
policies applicable to the system should take into consideration the specific characteristics and needs of the
organization.*

*When choosing a documentation system, the nurs-
ing leadership must be a key participant on the planning and implementation team. All systems, manual and
computerized, have strengths and weaknesses. A key
factor in implementing any system of documentation
is that it is used consistently and correctly as designed.
This will increase the credibility of the documentation,
and the probability that the documentation is valid and
reliable will be enhanced.*

*This chapter illustrates this point by discussing the
case of* Lama v. Borras (1994).

In this chapter, you will learn:

1. Key legal requirements of a documentation system
2. The importance of careful implementation to ensure that the selected system is used consistently in a correct manner
3. The consequences, as illustrated by the case of *Lama v. Borras*, of failure to correctly and consistently use the selected system of documentation

ESTABLISH LEGAL STANDARDS FOR ALL SYSTEMS OF DOCUMENTATION

Regardless of the system used to document a patient's medical care and treatment, the implementation plan must include the means to ensure that all users of the system understand the way the system works and are trained to use it correctly. In addition, the use and effectiveness of the system must be monitored so that problems can be identified and corrected in a timely manner. Organizations must also ensure that the documentation system is in compliance with all applicable laws and regulations.

In designing and using documentation systems, health care organizations should consider the various needs of the employees who will use the system. For example, if the organization uses traveling nurses, then the training of those nurses on the use of the system must address their unique needs. Traveling nurses can be exposed to many different systems as they work in various locations. Accordingly, their training must ensure that they understand your system and are consistently capable of using it correctly. The organization might consider employing only those traveling nurses who are versed and adept in the operation and use of their particular system (Brous, Boulay, & Burger, 2011).

════════════════════════════*FAST FACTS in a NUTSHELL*

Any system of documentation must be used consistently and correctly. This will increase the credibility, validity, and reliability of the documentation.

ENSURE CONSISTENT AND CORRECT USE OF THE SELECTED DOCUMENTATION SYSTEM

There are a number of different approaches to documentation. Whatever system an organization chooses to use, it must be consistently used to ensure that the system achieves the intended goals of documentation. In addition, where it can be shown that a system is consistently and correctly used, it is easier to establish that the data in the record are valid and reliable should questions arise later.

Case Review: *Lama v. Borras* (1994)

To illustrate this point, consider the case of *Lama v. Borras* (1994). The system of charting in this case was charting by exception (CBE). In this system, the practice is not to document routine care, but rather to document the exceptions to the norm. In this case, Mr. Lama underwent surgical repair by Dr. Borras. He developed a postoperative infection while still in the hospital. He spent months subsequently being treated for the infection, after which he brought a suit against the surgeon and the hospital, seeking compensation for the damages he incurred.

During his postoperative care on May 17, a nurse's note indicates that the bandage covering the surgical wound was "very bloody," a symptom which, according to expert testimony, indicates the possibility of infection. On May 18, the patient was experiencing pain at the surgical site, and on May 19, the documentation noted the bandage was "soiled again." On May 20, Lama began to experience severe discomfort in his back. At some point on May 21, an attending physician diagnosed an infection of the space between the vertebral discs, and initiated treatment.

In this case, the Court, and apparently the trial jury, were troubled that a more complete account of Lama's evolving condition was unavailable, and it wrote, "because the hospital instructed nurses to engage in 'charting by exception,' a system whereby nurses did not record qualitative observations for each of the day's three shifts, but instead made such notes only when necessary to chronicle important changes in a patient's condition . . ." (pp. 475–476). The court also noted in the record that the nurses did not always adhere to CBE, and that at times they used a narrative style as well.

The court noted that the Puerto Rico Department of Health regulations that were in force in 1986 required qualitative nurses' notes for each nursing shift. This could have been a basis for finding the hospital liable in this matter on grounds of noncompliance with regulation.

However, the court went further and opined that "it was entirely possible for the jury to conclude that the particular way in which the medical and nursing records were kept constituted evidence of carelessness in monitoring the patient . . . Perhaps the infection would have been reported and documented earlier [otherwise]" (*Lama v. Borras*, 1994, p. 477).

Among the important lessons from this case is the need to ensure that a charting system is used consistently as designed. In this case, such information might have added credibility that the nurses' observations of the wound were adequate and met the standard of care. Additionally, an organization must be aware of and in compliance with the regulatory requirements governing their operations. Although it was not the basis for the court's decision in this case, noncompliance with regulations can be the basis for an adverse finding in a malpractice suit.

SUMMARY

Documentation systems must meet legal requirements, and policies applicable to the system should take into consideration the specific characteristics and needs of the organization. All systems have strengths and weaknesses, and a key factor in implementing any system of documentation is that it must be used consistently and correctly as designed. The system chosen should be consistently and correctly used as this will increase its credibility and reliability. Proper implementation is important, as this will increase the credibility, reliability, and validity of the documentation that is entered into the system.

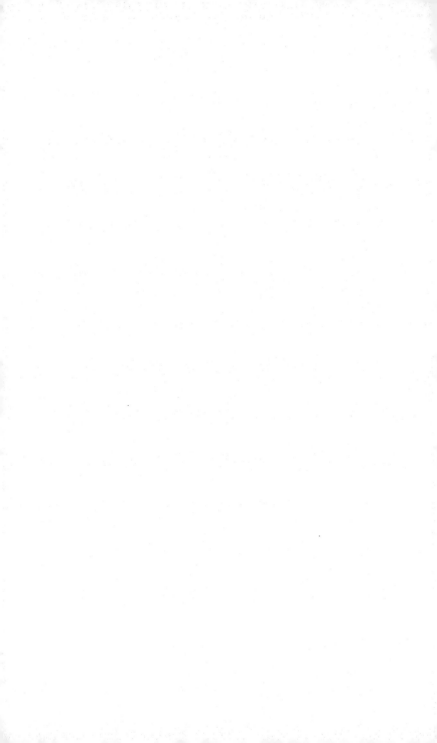

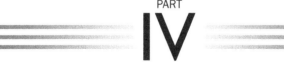

PART

IV

Informed Consent and Patient Rights

9

Requirements for Informed Consent

Diana C. Ballard

*The right to determine what will or will not be done to
one's person is long-standing in the law. The principle is
further shaped by ethical and moral considerations. A patient's right to accept or refuse treatment is enforced by
federal and state law, the Centers for Medicaid and Medicare Services (CMS), The Joint Commission (TJC), other
accrediting bodies, legal precedent, and ethical codes.*

*Nurses must understand the requirements of informed
consent and their own legal and ethical obligations with
regard to these principles.*

In this chapter, you will learn:

1. The required elements that constitute informed consent
2. The legal obligations of nurses, physicians, and hospitals with regard
   to informed consent
3. The sources of standards that determine whether the required
   elements of informed consent have been met

DEFINITION OF INFORMED CONSENT

Informed consent is not a document; it is a process. Informed consent can only be said to have occurred when the patient has sufficient information to make a reasoned, informed decision. Legally, this requires that the patient has been informed of the risks, benefits, alternatives, and costs associated with the treatment, test, or procedure for which he or she is giving his or her consent. This means that the patient must have received the necessary information and had the opportunity to ask questions and receive answers in order to arrive at an informed decision. Providers may not render the treatment, test, or procedure until such time as the patient has given his or her consent. Informed consent does not exist until a fully informed patient is able to make a rational choice about treatment or nontreatment. Thus, informed consent may be defined as the process by which a patient is adequately provided with all necessary information to participate in his or her health care decisions (Brous, 2011).

FAST FACTS in a NUTSHELL

Informed consent does not exist until a fully informed patient is able to make a rational choice about treatment or nontreatment.

THE DUTY TO PROVIDE INFORMED CONSENT

In most cases, the legal obligation to obtain informed consent belongs to the physician. This is due to the fact that in most cases, the physician is the person providing the care and treatment and thus is the person who is capable of providing the information that constitutes the required elements of informed consent.

Generally it is not within the scope of nursing practice to explain the risks, benefits, and alternatives to proposed treatment plans. However, given the evolving roles of advance practice nurses and other advanced practitioners, the legal framework of this requirement is changing. Since some jurisdictions have legally recognized this fact, new statutes may now permit advanced practitioners to obtain informed consent for procedures they perform. Since this is an evolving area, advance practice nurses should review the relevant law and regulation in the jurisdiction in which they practice for guidance on this important question (Brous, 2011).

NURSES' OBLIGATIONS WITH REGARD TO INFORMED CONSENT

Although in most cases the nurse does not have the legal duty to obtain informed consent, nurses do have obligations regarding consent. Nursing assessments include information about the patient's educational level, language proficiency, level of consciousness, and anxiety level. Even though patients may have concerns, they may not express those doubts or ask questions of their physicians. This can be due to a number of factors: language or cultural barriers, fear or intimidation, embarrassment, physical limitations such as diminished hearing or vision, or anxiety. Often the patient will ask the nurse questions about the contemplated treatment after the physician has left and the reality of the situation has become clearer to the patient. It is within the nurses' scope of practice to reinforce and clarify information for the patient. This is part of the health teaching role that is articulated in the Nurse Practice Act in the state in which the nurse practices and in the policies of the institution in which he or she works (Brous, 2011).

FAST FACTS in a NUTSHELL

It is within the nurse's scope of practice to reinforce and clarify information that a patient has received about the care and treatment he or she is to receive.

CAPACITY TO PROVIDE INFORMED CONSENT

Capacity means that an individual has the legal authority to provide consent for his or her own care and treatment. There are times when that legal authority does not rest with the person receiving the care and treatment, but rather with another person who has the legal authority to provide the informed consent on the patient's behalf.

For example, a minor does not have the legal authority to provide informed consent, and the parents or legal guardian must provide consent when needed. Other reasons for lack of capacity to consent to one's own care and treatment can be mental or physical impairment such that the individual cannot understand and comprehend the nature and consequences of providing consent.

The nurse must know who has the legal power of consent for minors or for patients without capacity. Nurses should not make any assumptions with regard to who has the legal power to consent for patients who lack such capacity. For example, a parent present with a child may not be the parent who has legal capacity to consent for a minor child, owing to a custody dispute or other legal proceeding. Likewise, a family member present with an incapacitated adult may not be the person who holds the legal authority to provide consent (Brous, 2011).

When a patient is admitted to a facility for care and treatment, admissions officers ascertain issues of legal authority, and this information is made part of the hospital record. If the nurse has any doubts or questions in this regard, he or she should seek clarification through normal administrative channels (Brous, 2011).

In an emergency situation, a physician may render treatment without consent if that is necessary to save life and if the time it would take to obtain consent would further jeopardize the patient's condition. Nurses should know the policies in their organization and seek administrative assistance with regard to any questions about the need to provide emergency care. This is discussed more fully in a later chapter.

FAST FACTS in a NUTSHELL

The nurse must know who has the legal power of consent for minors or for patients without capacity. It is risky to make any assumptions in this regard, and the nurse should take steps to confirm the identity of the person holding such authority.

NURSE AS PATIENT ADVOCATE

Nurses must identify any concerns or conflicts that a patient expresses to management and must understand that the patient has the right to withdraw previously given consent. The nurse has a legal obligation to advocate for patients in such circumstances. Nurses must advise the surgical or anesthesia team of the patient's concern, and it is essential that such information be properly documented in the medical record.

If nursing judgment suggests that the patient does not have the ability to understand the risks, benefits, and alternatives regarding the procedure, or that the patient has concerns that have not been addressed, that information must be communicated to the responsible providers before treatment is rendered (Brous, 2011).

======================*FAST FACTS in a NUTSHELL*

If the nurse has any doubts at all that the patient does not understand the risks, benefits, and alternatives or has concerns that have not been addressed with regard to treatment, he or she must communicate this to the responsible providers before any treatment is rendered.

SOURCES OF STANDARDS OF INFORMED CONSENT

Civil Lawsuits and Common Law

A patient may allege, in a civil lawsuit, that he or she received treatment without giving their consent. In such a suit, the patient may claim that he or she was not properly advised of complications, or did not have information as to the anticipated outcome of the procedure. He may claim that if he had complete information, he would not have consented to the procedure. The patient may allege that the provider failed to disclose risks that, if known, would have influenced her decision to consent to the treatment (Brous, 2011).

Decisions rendered by the court in such legal proceedings serve as precedent and thus influence future legal decisions. This type of law is also known as case law or common law and is law created by legal precedent.

STATUTES AND REGULATIONS

Statutes are laws created from action of legislatures. Regulations are laws created by administrative rulemaking. Nurses should know their organization's policies for informed consent, patient's rights, refusal of treatment, who can obtain informed consent, which procedures require consent, what constitutes an emergency, and the content of consent forms. The policies of an organization should, of course, reflect the standards and elements required by applicable statute and regulation.

For example, providers who participate in the Medicare program must agree to abide by Medicare's Conditions of Participation (CoP). The CoPs contain specific regulations with regard to informed consent. Similarly, state laws contain requirements in connection with informed consent.

One way that nurses can assist in confirming that the requirements of informed consent have been complied with is through careful and thorough documentation. Elements to include in documentation are that the patient understood and was able to repeat the information, or conversely, that the patient expressed concerns or reservations and that the physician and others, as appropriate, have been notified. In such cases, the nurse must be sure to follow the concerns to resolution. Documentation in such a situation should include which physician was notified and when, and what action followed. Seek administrative assistance if there are any lingering questions or issues that have not been resolved (Brous, 2011).

SUMMARY

Informed consent is not a document; it is a process. It can only be said to have occurred when the patient has information that is legally sufficient to demonstrate that the patient is able to make a reasoned and informed decision about his or her care or treatment. In general, the legal obligation to obtain informed consent belongs to the physician who is providing the care and treatment; however, given the evolving roles of advance practice nurses and other advanced practitioners, the legal framework of this requirement is changing. In true emergency situations and under certain conditions, treatment may be provided without consent.

10

High-Risk Areas Associated With Failure to Provide Informed Consent

Diana C. Ballard

> *Lack of consent is a common claim in malpractice suits. Even if the care itself was in conformance with proper standards of care, a claim of lack of consent can be made in a malpractice case. This is because failure to obtain consent is, by itself, a legal theory of negligence that allows for the recovery of damages (Brous, 2011).*

In this chapter, you will learn:

1. Areas of exposure to liability for failure to provide adequate informed consent
2. Ways to lessen exposure and potential liability to these high-risk areas

MALPRACTICE AND NEGLIGENCE

The most common reason a patient brings a lawsuit for lack of informed consent is a treatment complication. Specifically, the patient claims that he or she has suffered a complication about which he or she was not informed prior to agreeing to the treatment. The legal issue to be decided is whether or not the patient was advised of the possibility of the particular complication he or she has suffered (Brous, 2011).

Ordinary negligence is not an intentional act, and thus the patient does not have to show that the provider's actions were intentional. Rather, the patient must prove that the provider had a duty to provide reasonable care at the proper level of professional standards, failed to do so, and that because of that failure the patient sustained injury or damages.

The most valuable defense in such a case lies in the provider's documentation (Brous, 2011). The consent form itself should include a statement that the form was explained, that questions were answered to the patient's satisfaction, and that there were no blanks on the form at the time it was signed.

The physician or informing provider should also include notes in the record documenting the informed consent conversation that he or she has had with the patient. Such notes should include who was present in addition to the patient; that the nature of the procedure, alternatives, and risks were discussed; and that the patient appeared to comprehend and understand the information that was transmitted during the conversation. Providers are well advised to be as specific as they can be about the informed conversation documentation, as this may be an important record for the defense in the event of a legal challenge (Brous, 2011).

LICENSURE

Patients who decide to file a suit may also file a complaint with the professional licensing board. A complaint with a licensing board is an administrative process, and can occur whether or not a suit is filed in a court of law (Brous, 2011).

Licensing boards are obliged to investigate any complaint that is filed. On the basis of the finding of the board, the complaint may be dismissed and the case closed with no further action. Conversely, the board may find that a licensed provider has performed in a negligent manner, or engaged in professional misconduct, or practiced below an acceptable standard of care. Professional licensing boards also have the discretion to take action against the license of a physician, nurse, or other licensed provider, which can result in temporary or permanent license suspension. They may also limit practice under the individual's license or order remedial education (Brous, 2011).

Licensing boards have wide discretion in such matters. Further, the standard of proof in administrative matters is typically lower than in a court of law. The most common standard in these cases is preponderance of the evidence, which basically means that based on the evidence, it is more likely than not that professional misconduct has occurred.

BATTERY

An allegation that a patient was treated without giving consent can lead to a charge of battery. Battery is specifically defined under state laws, but in general it means an unauthorized touching or offensive contact. Unlike negligence, battery is an intentional act. If the patient also alleges that he or she was given misleading or false information, he or she may also be able to assert a claim of fraud (Brous, 2011).

DUTY TO NONPATIENT THIRD PARTIES

An interesting question arises when a patient who is treated by a physician causes harm to others due to side effects from the treatment. This situation can come up, for example, in a case in which a patient received medication that impairs his or her ability to drive and the patient ultimately causes an auto accident in which other persons are injured. The question is: Can the prescribing physician be held liable for the injuries sustained by those other persons?

A provider may be held responsible for injuries to third parties due to the failure to advise the patient of impairment caused by his or her medical condition or medication side effects.

This principle is illustrated in the case of *Coombes v. Florio* (2007). In this case, the mother of a 10-year-old child sued a physician who had prescribed numerous medications to a patient without advising him not to drive. The 75-year-old man lost consciousness while driving. The child was standing on the sidewalk when he was struck and killed by the man's car. On appeal, the court held that the physician was liable since he owed a duty of reasonable care to everyone foreseeably put at risk by the physician's failure to warn of the side effects of the patient's treatment. In this case, the court noted that the man was on numerous medications and that, considering the patient's age and health, it was foreseeable that the patient would suffer side effects that would impair his driving and an accident would result (p. 184).

Nurses should take great care in documenting instructions to patients regarding potential impairment from, among other things, medications, seizures, or other medical conditions. Policies should also be clear regarding the length of time a patient must be observed after being medicated, emerging from anesthesia, or receiving conscious sedation (Brous, 2011).

REDUCING EXPOSURE TO LIABILITY

The key to reducing exposure to liability for matters concerning informed consent is to take the time necessary to be sure the patient has the information necessary to make an informed decision. It is important to remember that informed consent is a process. It is not the signing of a form alone, nor is it an administrative procedure that can be delegated to a clerical worker who obtains the signature of a patient on a form.

The person obtaining the informed consent should be the person who is familiar with the patient's medical condition and is in a position to evaluate the patient's ability to understand what is being discussed. In most cases, this is the physician who is performing the procedure or administering the treatment. The practitioner providing the informed consent should be sure to advise the patient that there is a possibility a procedure may not produce the desired benefit. Documentation of the conversation should include any change in plan, such as incidental procedures or change in anesthesia, that may be required during the procedure. The documentation should also include specifics that were discussed, including a description of specific risks, benefits, and alternatives. Note should also be made of the patient's level of consciousness at the time of the discussion. If others were present at the discussion, those witnesses should be identified in the record. Nurses witnessing signatures should also document the patient's level of consciousness at the time the consent was signed (Brous, 2011).

The physician or nurse should not underestimate the value of a relationship with the patient. Having rapport with the patient helps to establish a positive relationship and instill trust, and promotes higher quality of communication. This positive environment is enhanced by ensuring that enough time is set aside for the informed consent discussion, so that the patient does not feel rushed or pressured. Patients should be comfortable in feeling that there is enough time for their questions to be answered (Brous, 2011).

===============*FAST FACTS in a NUTSHELL*

Do not underestimate the value of a relationship with the patient. Having rapport with the patient helps to establish a positive relationship and instill trust, and promotes higher quality of communication.

The patient's response to medication should also be documented in the record, to avoid later claims that the consent forms were signed while the patient was distracted from pain or impaired from narcotics. Notation should be made of the date and time the consent form was signed. If any written materials or diagrams were reviewed with the patient, copies of those items should be included in the medical record (Brous, 2011).

Organizations and providers differ in the design and content of forms used to document informed consent. Overall, the form should be written in language that is clear and understandable. The form is placed in the medical record prior to the procedure. The form should describe the procedure that the patient is to undergo, and the procedure that is actually done should not exceed any procedures that are mentioned or contemplated in the form. The form should be designed to provide evidence of a complete record of the information communicated to the patient. It may include a checklist of common risks and may have space for specific or additional risks that can be written in. The dated, timed, and witnessed consent form should contain a statement that the form contained no blanks when it was signed. This will help to avoid any suggestion that information was added after the form was signed. Language should be included in the form stating that it was read before being signed, that it was reviewed with the patient, and that the patient's questions were answered (Brous, 2011).

As has already been stated, informed consent is a process and not a form. The consent form that the patient signs should be an accurate and complete record of the conduct of that process.

In the event that there is a language barrier with the patient, an interpreter should be used to assist in communicating with the patient. The interpreter should be approved by the facility, and identified by last name in the record. It is generally not a good idea to use a family member or nonapproved staff member for such purposes, as there is no assurance that such a person would possess the necessary language skills or have the level of understanding needed to assist in the communication of medical information. Your facility should have a procedure in place to have approved resources available for assisting in these matters (Brous, 2011).

═══════════════════════════════════*FAST FACTS in a NUTSHELL*

Informed consent is a process and not a form. The consent form that the patient signs is the record of the conduct of that process.

EXCEPTIONS TO THE REQUIREMENT FOR INFORMED CONSENT

Emergency Situations

When treatment delays can result in loss of life, limb, or organ, providers may intervene under the theory of implied consent. Implied consent presumes that the patient would have consented in the emergency circumstance had he or she been able to do so. The law is based on what a reasonable person would have agreed to under the same or similar circumstances. Nurses should be aware of their organization's policies for situations in which it is not possible to obtain informed consent prior to providing urgently needed treatment. In addition, nurses should not hesitate to seek guidance from administration in these circumstances, so that they are not applying the policy in a situation on their own (Brous, 2011).

An organization's policies with regard to patient consent in emergency situations should address minors and patients without capacity. Documentation in these situations should include the provider's clinical impression of why emergency treatment is required and the potential consequences of a delay in treatment. The documentation should also specify steps, if any, that were taken to try and obtain informed consent from another designated person who may be in a position to provide consent when the patient cannot. This person is referred to as a proxy. In all situations, providers must avoid the appearance of labeling a situation as an emergency in order to carry out procedures without consent (Brous, 2011).

═══════════════════════════*FAST FACTS in a NUTSHELL*

In some emergency situations, consent may be assumed as a matter of law. Caregivers must make reasonable efforts to obtain consent and must never label a situation as an emergency in order to carry out procedures without consent.

Statutory or Legal Exceptions

There are some nonemergency situations where consent may be presumed as a matter of law. Laws for these types of situations vary by state, and nurses must be aware of the laws of their state. Many states allow blood alcohol levels to be obtained from patients being treated for motor vehicle accident injuries. In states where this is permitted, the driver is presumed to consent to such testing as a condition for maintaining a driver's license. Some states permit organ or tissue donation in the absence of an express refusal to donate. Still some other states require mandatory testing for certain diseases. Mental health laws in some states may allow for mandatory treatment or admission in the absence of patient consent (Brous, 2011).

Emancipation

In usual situations, the consent of a parent or legal guardian is required for treatment of a minor patient. There are times when a patient below the age of majority can provide consent or refusal for his or her own care or treatment, if he or she is considered under the law to be "emancipated." State laws vary in specifying conditions necessary for a minor to be deemed emancipated, and may include considerations such as military service, pregnancy, marriage, or high school graduation. Specific state laws also address treatments for which parental consent is not required and generally include reproductive issues, mental health intervention, addiction, and sexually transmitted diseases (Brous, 2011).

Substituted Judgment

As has already been discussed, informed consent requires that the person have decision-making capacity. If the person cannot understand what is being communicated, then he or she may be unable to consider the nature of the treatment, risks, alternatives, and benefits to the treatment. Many conditions can affect decision-making capacity: mental illness, extreme anxiety, altered level of consciousness, intoxication, or other factors. In some cases, it may be necessary to have the court appoint a guardian to make decisions for the incapacitated patient. In other cases, patients may have already planned for this eventuality by designating someone to make decisions on their behalf through the use of advance directives (Brous, 2011).

Therapeutic Privilege

In rare cases, a provider may avoid disclosing certain risks associated with a procedure if in his or her clinical opinion it is determined that it may be detrimental to the patient to disclose the information. This exception is appropriate only in very limited circumstances, and only when the provider believes that the patient may experience physical or emotional injury from the disclosure. If this exception is used, the provider must document the rationale for withholding the information. It is also advised that a provider seek input from an ethics committee, family members, or other appropriate resources when possible (Brous, 2011).

SUMMARY

Lack of consent is a common claim in malpractice suits. The failure to obtain informed consent is, by itself, a legal theory of negligence that allows for recovery of damages. A key to reducing exposure to liability for matters involving informed consent is to take the time necessary to be sure the patient has the necessary information to make an informed decision. Careful documentation of the content and nature of the informed consent discussion is vital. Nurses and providers should know who has the capacity to provide informed consent and should be familiar with conditions under which there may be exceptions to the requirement for informed consent. The most valuable defense in a case based on lack of informed consent may lie in the provider's documentation.

11

The Patient Self-Determination Act and Advance Directives

Diana C. Ballard

A person's right to make end-of-life decisions has developed over time and in concert with a number of landmark cases and legislative acts. In 1990, Congress enacted the Patient Self-Determination Act (PSDA) as part of the Omnibus Reconciliation Act of 1990 (PL 101–158). This legislation was intended to provide legal tools to assist individuals to exercise their constitutional right to determine their final health care (Brous, 2011).

In this chapter, you will learn:

1. The major requirements for hospitals and certain health providers under the Patient Self-Determination Act, including the use of advance directives

PATIENT SELF-DETERMINATION ACT

Effective December 1, 1991, the Patient Self-Determination Act (PSDA) required health care institutions receiving funding from Medicare or Medicaid to provide all patients who are 18 years of age or older with the following written information:

- The patient's rights under the law to participate in decisions about his or her medical care, including the right to accept or refuse treatments
- The patient's right under state law to complete advance directives, which would be documented in his or her medical records
- The health care provider's policies honoring these rights

Providers include hospitals, nursing homes, home health care providers, hospices, and health maintenance organizations, but not outpatient service providers or emergency medical personnel. The PSDA requires these health care providers to educate their staff and the community about advance directives. It prohibits hospital personnel from discriminating against patients on the basis of whether they have an advance directive; thus, patients must be informed that having an advance directive is not a prerequisite to receiving care (Brous, 2011).

Advance directives are documents in which a patient can give instructions about his or her health care and end-of-life choices in a situation in which he or she is unable to speak for himself or herself. Living wills and medical power of attorney documents are examples of advance directives (Brous, 2011).

Although providers must make treatment decisions within the patient's advance directive wishes, it must be carefully explained to patients with existing Do Not Resuscitate (DNR) orders that the team will intervene for correctable surgical or anesthesia problems even though the patients have DNR status. A distinction must be drawn between resuscitation and treatment of an acute episode (Brous, 2011).

════════════════════════════════ *FAST FACTS in a NUTSHELL*

Advance directives are documents in which a patient can give instructions about his or her health care and end-of-life choices that can be followed in a situation in which he or she is unable to speak for himself or herself.

High-profile cases such as those of Nancy Cruzan (Cruzan, 1988), Karen Ann Quinlan (Quinlan, 1976), and Terri Schiavo (Schiavo, 2005) highlight the conflicts that can occur with end-of-life decisions. Religious, spiritual, and personal value systems play an important role in the choice to continue or discontinue life support. Disagreements abound relative to concepts of privacy, constitutional rights, human dignity, individual versus state interests, guardianship issues, sanctity versus quality of life distinctions, interpretation of living wills and more, and these are intensely emotional subjects. Organizational ethics committees, Nurse Practice Acts, and the position papers of professional organizations may provide guidance for difficult cases (Brous, 2011).

Every state has living-will-type statutes or legislation that provide for the expression of one's right to self-determination. In addition, there are a number of living will documents that include the forms that one would use to express his or her advance directive wishes. It is important that such a document conforms to the requirements of the relevant laws of the state where a patient undergoes treatment. Many available forms are valid in multiple states.

One excellent document is the "Five Wishes Living Will," a living will form that has been disseminated by a group called Aging With Dignity. Five Wishes was originally introduced in 1996 as a Florida-only document, combining a living will and health care power of attorney in addition to addressing matters of comfort care and spirituality. With help from the American Bar Association's Commission on Law and Aging and leading medical experts, a national version of Five Wishes was introduced in 1988. The Five Wishes Living Will meets the legal requirements in 42 states and can be included in the other 8 states along with the state-required documents (Aging With Dignity, n.d.).

Five Wishes is available in 26 languages. For additional information about the Five Wishes Living Will, contact:

Aging With Dignity
http://www.agingwithdignity.org
Phone: (850) 681-2010 ext. 107
P.O. Box 1661, Tallahassee, Florida 32302

SUMMARY

A person's right to make end-of-life decisions has developed over time and in concert with a number of landmark cases and legislative acts. The PSDA, living will statutes, and case law have helped to provide the legal tools to assist individuals to exercise their constitutional right to determine their final health care. Advance directives allow patients to give instructions about their health care and end-of-life decisions that go into effect when they can no longer speak for themselves. Conflicts can occur with end-of-life decisions, and nurses can find guidance in dealing with such situations through their organization's policies and ethics committees, Nurse Practice Act, and position papers of professional organizations.

PART

V

Employment Law

12

The Employment Relationship

Paula DiMeo Grant

Part V: Employment Law will examine the following areas: The Employment Relationship, Ethical Obligations and Wrongful Discharge, and an Overview of Federal Workplace Laws. This chapter will focus on the relationship between employee and employer. The relationship gives rise to certain rights and responsibilities in the workplace. Three main categories of employment will be discussed. The elements necessary for a valid employment contract will be reviewed, as well as breach of contract, the remedies for breach of contract, and the meaning of "just cause" for termination. Employment contracts may be verbal or written. The employment-at-will doctrine will also be reviewed, and case examples will be cited to illustrate points of law.

In this chapter, you will learn to:

1. Identify three categories of employment
2. Name the elements of an employment contract
3. Describe "just cause" for termination
4. Discuss the ANA's workplace Bill of Rights

EMPLOYMENT CATEGORIES AND CONTRACTS

Three Categories of Employment Relations

There are three main categories of employment relations between an employee and an employer:

1. Employment at will
2. Fixed term or specified term
3. Independent contractor

Employment at Will

The employment-at-will doctrine gives the employer the right to terminate an employee for any or no reason in the absence of a law or contract restricting such act. Although this doctrine has been slowly eroded by statutory and case laws, employers have used it to terminate employees without liability. There are exceptions to this doctrine as addressed by the courts. An exception to this doctrine is later illustrated in the case of *Toussaint v. Blue Cross, Blue Shield* (1980) (Grant & Vecchione, 2011).

Fixed-Term or Specified-Term Employment

Fixed- or specified-term employment is one that usually provides the employee with a written contract for a specified period of time for employment. Certain employment contracts for work that cannot be performed within 1 year are required to be in writing, and signed by the person to be charged, to comply with the "statute of frauds" in order to be enforceable.

Independent Contractor

An independent contractor is an individual hired to do a certain task or tasks, but is left free to determine how to accomplish them. There are certain factors set forth in the law to distinguish this type of employment from the others, such as: (a) employer's right to control, (b) the job skills, (c) the employee's length of service, (d) method of payment, and (e) the intent of the parties. The Internal Revenue Service (IRS) will look to the relationship of the parties' behavioral and financial control to determine whether the relationship is one of independent contractor. It is important for the parties to have a clear understanding of this category of employment for income tax and liability purposes (Grant & Vecchione, 2011).

The Employment Contract

A valid contract contains three essential elements: (1) an offer, (2) acceptance, and (3) consideration. For example, an employer makes a job offer to a nurse; the nurse will either accept the job offer or reject it. If the job offer is accepted, there will be consideration or compensation given to the nurse by the employer for work perfomed. In order for the contract to be valid, there must be mutual understanding or mutual assent to the terms and conditions agreed upon by the parties. Contract elements are not always easy to determine, especially when they are not in writing. A contract that is not in writing is sometimes referred to as an implied contract, which may be established by an employee handbook or manual.

The employee handbook or manual distributed to employees contains employment policies and procedures as well as standards to follow. In some cases, courts have determined that employers are bound by the terms set forth in the manual. The leading case illustrating this principle was *Toussaint v. Blue Cross, Blue Shield* (1980).

CASE EXAMPLE

Wrongful Termination Claim

Toussaint v. Blue Cross & Blue Shield (1980)

Issue: Whether or not the language in the employment manual was deemed to form an implied contract of employment.

Plaintiff Toussaint was employed for a period of 5 years as a middle management employee before his termination. His employer, Blue Cross & Blue Shield, considered him an "at-will" employee, which it believed gave it the right to terminate him for any or no reason. Following termination, the plaintiff brought a wrongful discharge claim against his employer. The facts reveal that at the time of hiring, Toussaint was given an employment manual that, among other provisions, contained a "just cause" for termination clause. The manual also provided for disciplinary procedures for termination that apparently were not followed in this matter. Toussaint also claimed to have been given job security assurances by a Blue Cross representative at the time of hiring. The Michigan Supreme Court found in Toussaint's favor under the theory of implied contract, based on the language in the employment manual.

COURT'S DECISION: The court based its rationale on the fact that an employer will be denied its right to terminate an at-will employee for any reason whatsoever if the employer chooses to publish an employee handbook with a "just cause" for termination. The employee manual, in this case, was deemed to form an implied contract for employment. At the time, this landmark decision became a national trend. Since this case was decided, Michigan has clarified and modified the employment-at-will doctrine. Today, the doctrine varies from state to state.

Just Cause for Termination

In some instances, as in Toussaint, decisions of the courts may turn on the language in the handbook, which provides for termination of an employee only for "just cause," or good reason, thus preventing the employer from using the employment-at-will doctrine, as previously discussed. The employment contract governs both performance and conduct in the workplace. A written agreement allows the parties to have a better understanding of their rights and responsibilities in the workplace. "Just cause" for termination clauses are often included for managerial or nurse practitioners or both in written employment contracts. Each termination case is decided on its own merits and may not have a favorable outcome for the employee.

══════════════════════════ *FAST FACTS in a NUTSHELL*

An employment contract consists of three elements: an offer, acceptance, and consideration.

══════════════════════════ *FAST FACTS in a NUTSHELL*

The employment-at-will doctrine gives the employer the right to terminate an employee for any or no reason in the absence of a law or contract restricting such an act.

Collaborative Agreements

In some instances, there may be a written collaborative agreement between a physician and a nurse practitioner, as required by state law. In some states, these agreements may also be required for reimbursement purposes. Collaborative agreements should clearly delineate the responsibilities of the nurse practitioners and physicians, indicating the scope of nursing practice, including prescriptive authority when warranted. Employment contracts that are in writing should provide a clear understanding of the terms and conditions agreed upon by the parties, thus minimizing or eliminating misunderstandings.

Collective Bargaining Agreements

A collective bargaining agreement is "a contract between employer and a labor union regulating employment conditions, wages, benefits and grievances" (*Black's Law Dictionary*, 2010, p. 240). It is imperative that all nurses covered by these agreements and the management personnel supervising them know and fully understand the terms and conditions contained in the provisions of the agreement. The rights and responsibilities of the employees and the employer have been negotiated and ratified by the membership and reduced to writing. The collective bargaining agreement provides the legal framework for the employment relationship (Grant & Vecchione, 2011).

Breach of Contract

Once a valid contract is formed, it may be breached by either the employee or employer. A breach of contract occurs when the terms and conditions of employment have been violated by either party. Many breach of contract claims are instituted by employees for wrongful discharge. The remedies for breach of contract vary and may include monetary damages and reinstatement of employment.

It is common to have a combination of legal theories with breach of contract claims such as discrimination. Federal antidiscrimination statutes will be addressed in a later chapter.

===============*FAST FACTS in a NUTSHELL*

A collective bargaining agreement is "a contract between employer and a labor union regulating employment conditions, wages, benefits and grievances" (*Black's Law Dictionary*, 2010).

American Nurses Association: Workplace Bill of Rights

In 2001, the American Nurses Association (ANA) adopted a Bill of Rights for registered nurses (RNs). The ANA believes that to maximize the contributions that nurses make in society, it is necessary to protect the autonomy and dignity of nurses in the workplace, as embodied in the Bill of Rights. Those rights include the right to practice in accordance with professional standards and legally authorized scopes of nursing practice in accordance with the ANA Code of Ethics. According to this bill, nurses have a right to negotiate conditions of employment and safe working environment for themselves and patients. While these rights are not legally binding, they can be useful in forming the basis for employment contracts, including collective bargaining agreements (Grant & Vecchione, 2011).

Workplace Tools

Exhibit 12.1 is a list of workplace tools that can provide guidance for nurses in the clarification of issues that may arise in their employment settings and in the formulation of employment policies and procedures (Grant & Vecchione, 2011, p. 132).

Exhibit 12.1   Workplace Tools for Nurses

1. Nurse Practice Acts
2. Employment contracts
3. Collective bargaining agreements
4. Employment manuals or handbooks
5. Employment policies and procedures
6. Standards of nursing practice
7. ANA Code of Ethics for Nurses with Interpretive Statements
8. ANA Bill of Rights for Nurses
9. ANA Workplace Position Statements
10. Nursing Specialty Organizations Position Statements

═══════════════════════════*FAST FACTS in a NUTSHELL*

In 2001, the ANA adopted a workplace Bill of Rights for RNs.

SUMMARY

The demand for highly skilled registered nurses in the workplace will continue to grow. Employment contracts, collective bargaining agreements, employment policies and procedures, and employment manuals provide guidance regarding nurses' rights and responsibilities in the workplace. Nurses should also remain mindful of the Nurse Practice Act and the Code of Ethics. The employment relationship between employer and employee gives rise to certain rights and responsibilities as well as remedies for breach of contract.

The ANA Bill of Rights for Nurses is supportive of nurses in the workplace and may be used as a guide in the development of workplace policies and procedures.

13

Ethical Obligations and Wrongful Discharge

Paula DiMeo Grant

This chapter will focus on ethical dilemmas in the work-place. Professional ethical codes of conduct are sometimes in conflict with employment policies and procedures when addressing ethical dilemmas. Wrongful discharge cases will be used to illustrate salient points regarding ethical obligations. Ethical concepts in nursing practice will be explored. The American Nurses Association (ANA) Code of Ethics with Interpretive Statements defines the ethical parameters for nursing practice and forms the framework for nurses responding to ethical dilemmas.

In this chapter, you will learn to:

1. Identify ethical concepts in nursing practice
2. Discuss the purpose of the ANA Code of Ethics for Nurses
3. Discuss ethical dilemmas in the workplace and wrongful discharge from employment

ETHICAL CONCEPTS AND DILEMMAS

Ethical Concepts in Nursing Practice

1. **Autonomy:** The ethical concept of individual autonomy is the right of the individual to make decisions regarding his or her own medical care.
2. **Justice:** This ethical principle is based upon fairness to all people and equal access to health care for all people.
3. **Fidelity:** The ethical concept of fidelity includes faithfulness to commitments made to self and others. It also includes accountability and fulfilling contractual obligations.
4. **Beneficence:** The ethical concept of beneficence obliges you to do good for your patients, taking into consideration the patient's personal beliefs and that of family when necessary.
5. **Nonmaleficence:** This ethical principle is to do no harm, either intentionally or unintentionally.
6. **Veracity:** This ethical concept includes the patient's right to know truthful information. Health care providers are not to deceive or mislead patients.
7. **Best Interests:** The ethical principle of best interests takes into consideration what the individual has expressed either formally or informally (Grant, 2011).

These key concepts in ethics have been included and expanded in the nine provisions of the ANA Code of Ethics for Nurses.

ANA Code of Ethics for Nurses

The ANA Code of Ethics for Nurses with Interpretive Statements (2001) describes the ethical obligations and duties of nurses, and assists nurses with the application of ethical principles in the delivery of patient care. The Code contains nine provisions and serves the following purposes:

1. It states the ethical obligations of nurses in the delivery of patient care
2. It identifies ethical obligations that are nonnegotiable
3. It is an expression of these obligations to the profession and to society as a whole

Ethical Dilemmas in the Workplace

There are times when workplace situations between employee and employer present ethical dilemmas that may conflict with Professional Ethical Codes of Conduct. The ANA Code of Ethics for Nurses (2001), Provision 6, states: "The nurse participates in establishing, maintaining and improving healthcare environments and conditions of employment conducive to the provision of high quality care and consistent with the value of the profession through individual and collective action." Provision 3 of the Code further states: "The nurse promotes, advocates for and strives to protect the health, safety and rights of the parties" (ANA, 2001). Nurses face many challenges in the delivery of optimal patient care in light of the increased demands placed on them as a result of rapid changes in the health care system. The delivery of safe patient care continues to be paramount, irrespective of these demands.

═══════════════════════════*FAST FACTS in a NUTSHELL*

The ANA Code of Ethics defines the ethical parameters for nursing practice. It also provides guidance to nurses faced with ethical dilemmas.

Wrongful Discharge Cases

It is common to have a combination of contract and tort theories and/or charges of discrimination in wrongful discharge cases. Careful analysis of the facts by competent counsel is necessary when termination occurs to ascertain whether a valid claim for wrongful discharge exists. The following three cases illustrate examples of workplace situations involving ethical issues and wrongful discharge claims (Grant & Vecchione, 2011, pp. 129, 130).

CASE EXAMPLES

Doctor Refuses to Work on New Drug for Ethical Reasons

Pierce v. Ortho Pharmaceuticals (N.J. 1980)

Issue: Whether Dr. Pierce was wrongfully terminated from employment for refusing an assignment because of an ethical belief.

Dr. Pierce was an employee of Ortho Pharmaceuticals in New Jersey. She was assigned to work on a new drug product by her employer. Dr. Pierce refused the assignment for ethical reasons because she believed a safer drug that would be more beneficial to the public could soon be developed. She was terminated by her employer for refusing the assignment. She brought a lawsuit for wrongful termination.

COURT'S DECISION: The court ruled in favor of the employer, Ortho Pharmaceuticals. However, the court also recognized that employees owe a special duty to abide not only by federal and state laws but also by the recognized Codes of Ethics promulgated by their professions. In this case that "special duty" was not deemed by the court to fall into the category of the public policy exception to the at-will rule. Clearly, this situation presented an ethical dilemma for the employee that the court recognized, yet it ended unfavorably for the employee. Since the Pierce case was decided, the New Jersey legislature has enacted a whistleblower statute and the Conscientious Employee Protection Act of 1986 (CEPA; Standler, 2000). Although there are no guarantees of outcome when a lawsuit is filed, this case might have had a different outcome if these laws were in place at the time of the suit.

Nurse Questions Consent Form

Kraus v. New Rochelle Hospital (N.Y. 1995)

Issue: Whether a nurse was wrongfully discharged for questioning informed consent forms.

This lawsuit was brought by a vice president of nursing against her employer for wrongful discharge and other claims. The facts reveal that the plaintiff identified problems with informed consent forms that were obtained by a physician. She presented her concerns regarding the informed consent forms to the hospital's administrator. The hospital's medical board was notified about the complaint made by the vice president of nursing. A meeting with the hospital's medical board was subsequently held to discuss the issue. The outcome of the meeting was a "vote of no confidence" for the vice president of nursing by the medical board. As a result of the board's vote, the nurse's employment was terminated even though she had above-average performance evaluations. A wrongful termination suit was commenced, and there was a trial by jury.

COURT'S DECISION: The jury ruled in favor of Nurse Kraus and awarded her damages of US$703,250 for loss of income and fringe benefits. In addition, she was awarded US$587,200 in legal fees and expenses for her wrongful discharge suit. The employer appealed the decision. The Court of Appeals reduced the award and also ordered that she be reinstated to her former position as vice president of nursing.

Nurse Refuses to Float

Winkleman v. Beloit Memorial Hospital (Wisc. 1992)

Issue: Whether or not the nurse was wrongfully discharged for her refusal to float to an area where she felt unqualified.

Nurse Winkleman had 40 years of experience in maternity and neonatal care and was employed by Beloit Memorial Hospital. As a result of short staffing, she was ordered by the hospital to "float" and provide nursing care to postoperative and geriatric patients. She refused to float on the grounds that she was not qualified to work in those areas of nursing because her expertise was in maternity and neonatal care. The hospital interpreted her refusal to float as a voluntary resignation from employment. Winkleman filed a suit for wrongful discharge. She had a trial by jury.

COURT'S DECISION: A jury in Wisconsin found that the nurse had been wrongfully discharged for her refusal to float to an area of the hospital where she did not feel competent. She was awarded US$39,344 in lost earnings. The employer appealed the decision to the Supreme Court of Wisconsin, which affirmed the decision of the lower court.

The three cases illustrated are a small sampling of the kinds of ethical dilemmas that led to wrongful discharge that nurses and other health care providers faced in the workplace. In the Pierce case, the court, although it ruled in favor of the employer (hospital) and not the employee (physician) for refusal to work on a new drug for ethical reasons, also recognized that the employer owes a special duty to abide by recognized codes of ethics as promulgated by the profession. Since Pierce was decided in 1980, New Jersey has enacted laws to protect the employee in similar situations. Other states have also enacted whistleblower statutes to protect employees from wrongful discharge and retaliation for reporting substandard care or for refusing to carry out unethical practices.

═══════════════════════════*FAST FACTS in a NUTSHELL*

There are times when workplace situations present ethical dilemmas that conflict with professional codes of ethics.

Winkler County Nurses

A recent and landmark case involving two Texas nurses is also instructive regarding ethical obligations. After reporting a physician to the Texas Medical Board for substandard care, the nurses were indicted on criminal charges and subsequently were terminated from employment at a small Texas hospital where they had been employed for many years. After several years of litigation, which began in 2009, these nurses prevailed. This case has become known as the "Winkler County Nurses" (Texas Nurses Association, 2012).

═══════════════════════════*FAST FACTS in a NUTSHELL*

Ethical dilemmas in the workplace can sometimes lead to wrongful discharge of employees.

SUMMARY

Whereas the Nurse Practice Acts define the scope of nursing practice for nurses, it is the Code of Ethics for Nurses with Interpretive Statements that defines the ethical parameters of practice for nurses. The Code serves to identify the obligations of nurses in carrying out their duties, and those obligations as expressed are nonnegotiable. The ethical concepts discussed in this chapter are embodied in the Code. Nurses will continue to be challenged by the ethical dilemmas they face while delivering health care in this changing health care environment.

14

Federal Workplace Laws

Paula DiMeo Grant

The federal laws and regulations that govern the workplace are numerous and varied. This chapter will describe a sampling of these laws, some of which date back more than 100 years. These laws were enacted to protect job applicants and employees from various types of discrimination in the workplace. In recent years, antidiscrimination laws have been more inclusive of protected classes. In many instances, discrimination claims are brought in conjunction with breach of contract claims. The federal antidiscrimination laws discussed in this chapter may not apply to all employers.

In this chapter, you will learn to:

1. Identify federal antidiscrimination laws
2. Describe the role of the Equal Employment Opportunity Commission

OVERVIEW OF FEDERAL ANTIDISCRIMINATION LAWS

There are a vast array of antidiscrimination laws, some of which are listed below:

1. The Civil Rights Act of 1866 (Section 1981)
2. The Civil Rights Act of 1871 (Section 1983)
3. Title VII of the Civil Rights Act of 1964 (42 U.S.C. Sections 1981, 1983, and 2000 [e] et seq.)
4. The Age Discrimination in Employment (ADEA), 29 U.S.C. (Section 621)
5. The Americans with Disabilities Act (ADA), 42 U.S.C. (Section 1201)
6. The Family and Medical Leave Act (FMLA), 29 U.S.C. (Section 2601) (Grant & Vecchione, 2011).

Civil Rights Act of 1866 (Section 1981)

The oldest of the civil rights statutes is Section 1981 of the Civil Rights Act. It broadly protects individuals against all forms of racial and national origin discrimination in the making and enforcing of contracts.

Civil Rights Act of 1871 (Section 1983)

The Civil Rights Act of 1871, Section 1983, applies only to state government officials or those acting under the "color of law." It is broad in its scope and protects against racial discrimination and any violation of constitutional rights. The following are case examples of court decisions involving this act.

CASE EXAMPLES OF THE CIVIL RIGHTS ACT OF 1871 (SECTION 1983) (Grant & Vecchione, 2011, p. 109)

Weyandt v. Mason's Stores, Inc. (1968)

A Pennsylvania court, in the case of *Weyandt v. Mason's Stores, Inc.* (1968), decided that there was no Section 1983 claim against the store manager or detective for a wrongful shoplifting arrest. The law allowed a store manager to detain a person for shoplifting until the police arrived, but that did not mean he was acting under the color of state law. The manager was not acting as an officer himself. Similarly, just because the state issued detective licenses to security employees, it does not mean they were not acting "under color of law"; they were not acting on behalf of the state.

Carter v. Norfolk Community Hospital Association, Inc. (1985)

A state-owned or state-run hospital or health care facility might violate Section 1983 by failing to provide due process before making an employment decision or by discriminating on the basis of sex or race, but Section 1983 would not apply to a private hospital. This is so even if the hospital receives Medicaid or Medicare payments and, therefore, is required to comply with state regulations of those programs. For example in Carter, the court held that there was no Section 1983 violation for termination of physician's professional privileges.

Wong v. Stripling (1989) and Sarin v. Samaritan Health Care Center (1987)

In the case of *Wong v. Stripling* (1989), the court decided that revocation of hospital privileges is not "state action" even when state legislation authorized revocation and made courts available for review of procedural fairness of revocation. Therefore, there was no section 1983 violation. In *Sarin v. Samaritan Health Care Center* (1987), the revocation of privileges was not state action even when the hospital was licensed and regulated by the state, and the court decided in favor of the health care center.

In each of the above cases, the facts did not support a finding of a violation of the statute.

Nieto v. Kappoor (2001)

Nonetheless, Section 1983 does apply to those working for state or federal hospital systems as this case illustrates. Nieto was a case of harassment by the medical director of a public hospital and was thus found to be covered by Section 1983, as the public hospital was a state actor. It covers a much broader range of activities than Section 1981, including both race and sex discrimination.

Title VII of the Civil Rights Act of 1964

Title VII of the Civil Rights Act of 1964 prohibits discrimination based upon race, color, religion, national origin, or sex and has been referred to as the premier antidiscrimination statute of the federal government. It applies to employers with 15 or more employees. Sexual discrimination is prohibited by Title VII. This includes the creation of a sexually harassing environment for discrimination based upon sex. To prevail in a case of sexual harassment, a plaintiff must prove that:

1. He or she belongs to a protected class
2. He or she was subjected to unwelcome sexual harassment
3. The harassment was based upon sex (*Meritor Savings Bank v. Vinson*, 1986)

Employers must take affirmative steps to monitor and remove discrimination. As a general rule, employers are expected to provide sexual harassment training to all management personnel and to have policies and procedures in place for reporting sexual harassment. Should a lawsuit based upon sexual harassment be brought, courts will scrutinize policies and procedures and educational training of staff. Employers have a duty to prevent sexual harassment in the workplace.

The Age Discrimination in Employment Act

The Age Discrimination in Employment Act (ADEA) became effective in 1967 and prohibits discrimination based upon age of persons aged 40 and older. There are exceptions to this act, which include firefighters and police. In addition, it does not apply to employers with fewer than 20 employees or to the federal government. In the event that age and infirmity are the reasons why a person is no longer capable of performing the required job responsibilities, the ADEA does not mandate retention of the employee (Grant & Vecchione, 2011).

The Americans with Disabilities Act

In 1992, the Americans with Disabilities Act (ADA) became effective; the basic premise was that if jobs can be done by persons with disabilities, those jobs should be made available to them. This act requires that employers make reasonable accommodations to employees with disabilities to assist the employees with essential job responsibilities. Disability is defined broadly by this act. It includes: (a) a physical or mental impairment that substantially limits one or more major life activities of such individual; (b) a record of such impairment; or (c) being regarded as having such an impairment (42 U.S.C. Section 12102). "Reasonable accommodation is a modification or adjustment to the job or work environment that enables a worker or applicant to perform essential job functions" (Grant & Vecchione, 2011, p. 113).

The Family and Medical Leave Act

The Family and Medical Leave Act (FMLA) was enacted in 1993. Its purpose is to grant up to 12 weeks of unpaid leave to an employee experiencing certain family situations, such as the birth or adoption of a child or a serious health condition of the employee or spouse, child, or parent needing care. The employer is required to reinstate the employee to employment following the leave of absence. Specific conditions must be met before qualifying for this type of leave of absence. The law applies to employers with 50 or more employees, and there is a requirement that the employee must have worked a minimum of 1 year (Grant & Vecchione, 2011).

==================*FAST FACTS in a NUTSHELL*

There are a vast array of federal antidiscrimination laws, some of which date back more than 100 years.

ROLE OF EQUAL EMPLOYMENT OPPORTUNITY COMMISSION IN DISCRIMINATION CLAIMS

The Equal Employment Opportunity Commission (EEOC) is a federal agency that enforces the federal employment discrimination laws. These laws have a far-reaching effect because they are applied on a national level. EEOC offices are located nationwide. This agency has the authority to investigate charges of discrimination against employers that are covered by the laws, and issue "right-to-sue" letters to claimants bringing charges against employers. The agency may litigate or mediate claims on behalf of claimants. There are strict time frames in which to file EEOC claims. Employees who believe that their employment rights have been violated as described in the federal antidiscrimination laws that fall under the EEOC's jurisdiction may file a claim of discrimination with that agency. Questions should be addressed to competent counsel and/or the EEOC. There are instances when similar causes of action are covered by state statutes (Grant & Vecchione, 2011).

FAST FACTS in a NUTSHELL

The Equal Employment Opportunity Commission is the agency that enforces certain federal employment discrimination laws in the United States. It has the authority to investigate and address claims brought before the agency.

SUMMARY

This chapter provides an overview of the federal antidiscrimination laws to protect the U.S. worker in the workplace. Many of these laws apply to health care employers in this country. Violations of these laws can occur when employers engage in prohibited discrimination or take retaliatory action against employees for exercising protected rights. The EEOC has offices nationwide and is the agency charged with investigating violations of some of these antidiscrimination laws. In some instances, the EEOC will mediate or litigate claims on behalf of claimants or employees bringing charges against employers. In the event an employee suspects discrimination or retaliation in the workplace, a consultation with competent counsel to explore possible remedies may be in order.

Organization and Business Law: Topics for Nurses

15

Entity Types and Personal Liability for Owners

Diana C. Ballard

Corporate law includes laws and regulations governing the legal entities that may be formed to conduct business, and describes the attributes of the various structures. Nurses can benefit from knowledge of this area of the law in order to understand the operation of the organization they are affiliated with. In addition, many nurses are interested in starting their own business, and in such cases this information is invaluable in order to understand the legal methods of obtaining or filing required documents, and what other documents may be required, such as charters, articles of incorporation, or other legal filings or approvals (Ballard, Mitchell-Stoddard, & Radney, 2011).

There are a number of entities a nurse can choose to operate, and knowledge of the major attributes of each will assist the nurse in making an informed and appropriate choice. Nurses considering formation of an entity for the purpose of conducting business should seek advice of counsel experienced in this area of the law, as well as other professional business advisors as needed (Ballard, Mitchell-Stoddard, & Radney, 2011).

In this chapter, you will learn:

1. The types of entities that can be formed for the purpose of conducting business
2. The basic differences among the major types of entities

CORPORATIONS

A corporation is the most common form of business organization. A corporation is a legal entity or structure created under the authority of the laws of a state, consisting of a person or group of persons who become shareholders. The existence of a corporation is considered to be separate and distinct from that of its members, and the corporation has certain rights separate from those of its owners. Incorporation is the process of forming or becoming a corporation. The process of incorporation gives the company a separate legal standing from its owners, and protects its owners from being personally liable in the event that the company is sued. There are different tax implications for different types of corporations, which include the C corporations and S corporations, and tax-exempt versus taxable corporations (Ballard, Mitchell-Stoddard, & Radney, 2011).

Because a corporation is an entity considered separate and distinct from its members, a corporation itself can enter into contracts, sue and be sued, pay taxes separately from its owners, and can carry out actions necessary to conduct business. A corporation is also liable for its own debts and obligations. As a result, and providing that the corporate formalities are followed, the corporation's owners (the shareholders) enjoy limited liability and are legally shielded from the corporation's liabilities and debts (Ballard, Mitchell-Stoddard, & Radney, 2011).

Once formed, a corporation will continue to exist until such time as it is formally dissolved by the shareholders,

CHAPTER 15 ENTITY TYPES AND PERSONAL LIABILITY FOR OWNERS

merged with another business, or dissolved by state government for administrative reasons. Corporations are subject to the laws of the state where they are incorporated and to the laws of any other state in which the corporations conduct business (Ballard, Mitchell-Stoddard, & Radney, 2011).

=======================*FAST FACTS in a NUTSHELL*

Nurses considering formation of an entity for the purpose of conducting a business should seek advice of counsel as well as consulting other professional business advisors experienced in this area of the law.

TYPES OF CORPORATIONS

C Corporations

C corporations are corporations that are taxed separately from the shareholders, which means that the corporation itself pays taxes on net taxable income. The C corporation does not pass on business losses to the shareholders. The C corporation pays taxes on its taxable income before making distribution to its shareholders (Ballard, Mitchell-Stoddard, & Radney, 2011).

S Corporations

S corporations are corporations that elect to pass corporate income, losses, deductions, and credit through to their shareholders for federal income tax purposes. This permits shareholders of S corporations to report their share of corporate income and losses on their personal tax returns. This allows S corporations to avoid double taxation, which would be tax assessed on the corporate entity as well as tax paid on the income of the individual (Ballard, Mitchell-Stoddard, & Radney, 2011).

To qualify for S corporation status, a corporation must meet certain requirements, some of which are listed in the following:

- The corporation must be a domestic corporation, which means that it is formed in the state in which the shareholder resides.
- The corporation must meet the applicable requirements for numbers and type of shareholders.
- The corporation must be of a type that is eligible to be formed as an S corporation.

For-Profit and Not-for-Profit Corporations

The primary goal of for-profit corporations is to earn a profit and distribute such profit to shareholders. They can be privately held or publicly owned. Public companies trade on public markets, and shares of the company can be purchased, so the purchasers or shareholders share in the profits or losses of the company (Ballard, Mitchell-Stoddard, & Radney, 2011).

A not-for-profit corporation (also referred to as nonprofit, both terms being used interchangeably in this chapter) is a corporation that is formed and exists to carry out educational, charitable, or religious purposes. It is an organization incorporated under state laws and generally approved by both the state's Secretary of State and its taxing authority. Based on the type of nonprofit corporation and the purpose for which it is created, application may also be made to the Internal Revenue Service (IRS) for income tax exemption and other beneficial tax treatment. Note that state and federal tax treatments are applied for separately, and approval of one does not necessarily confer approval from the other (Ballard, Mitchell-Stoddard, & Radney, 2011).

The existence of not-for-profits is based on the fact that the organizations are operated exclusively for religious, charitable, scientific, or educational purposes. Ultimately, the community is to receive a benefit in return for the government's decision to allow the nonprofit to receive preferential tax treatment. Not-for-profit hospitals are usually organized under section 501(c)(3) of the Internal Revenue Code and are exempt from federal income taxes. Exemption from state taxes is not automatic and must be requested from the state taxing authority (Ballard, Mitchell-Stoddard, & Radney, 2011).

Nonprofit hospitals, for example, are not precluded from paying employees, managers, physicians, or others for their services; however, they are under more scrutiny to ensure that payments for services are not detrimental to the community. In fact, the incorporators, officers, or trustees of such an entity do not receive any financial benefits. Rather, any earnings from a not-for-profit entity are used to further the goals of its educational, charitable, scientific, or religious purpose (Ballard, Mitchell-Stoddard, & Radney, 2011).

Unlike a for-profit corporation, a not-for-profit corporation does not have shareholders. It is formed by incorporators and has a board of directors and officers. These incorporators, directors, and officers may not receive a distribution of (any money from) profits, but officers and management may be paid reasonable salaries for services to the corporation. Upon dissolution, which is disbanding or ceasing the existence of a not-for-profit corporation, its assets must be distributed to an organization existing for similar purposes under the cy pres doctrine. The French words *cy pres*, literally translated, mean "as close as possible"; therefore, the assets of a dissolved not-for-profit entity must be distributed to an organization operating for similar, or "as close as possible," purposes (Ballard, Mitchell-Stoddard, & Radney, 2011).

In order for contributions to a not-for-profit corporation to be deductible to the donor as charitable gifts on federal income taxes, the corporation must submit a detailed application for an IRS ruling confirming that the corporation is established for one of the specific not-for-profit purposes spelled out in the Internal Revenue Code. Not every tax-exempt entity will fit this requirement, so a donor must verify the specifics enabling a deduction for certain contributions (Ballard, Mitchell-Stoddard, & Radney, 2011).

Professional Corporations

A professional corporation (PC) is a corporation formed specifically for the purpose of conducting a profession that requires licensure to practice, such as nurses, physicians, attorneys, and dentists, to name a few. Most states provide for such PCs under special statutes that allow the corporation to operate under the direction of professionals in the discipline for which the corporation is formed. However, state laws vary, and nurses and other licensed professionals should check the laws in their state to determine which disciplines are eligible for this type of entity. In addition, there may be specific provisions governing whether a nurse can form a PC with another professional discipline, such as a physician. For these reasons, the nurse should seek advice of counsel in considering such issues (Ballard, Mitchell-Stoddard, & Radney, 2011).

A key point is that, unlike other types of corporations, a professional corporation does not provide a shield from liability for any professional negligence (malpractice) by the licensed professionals. This means that professional practitioners will be personally liable for any negligent acts occurring in the practice of their profession, despite the fact that they have formed the corporation (Ballard, Mitchell-Stoddard, & Radney, 2011).

SOLE PROPRIETORSHIP

Sole Proprietorship

The sole proprietorship is the simplest business form for an individual to utilize. A sole proprietor owns an unincorporated business as the sole owner. The business form can be established quickly and easily, as there is no necessity to file any documents with the state. (However, it should be noted that there may be other required filings and approval to consider based on the nature of the business to be carried out, such as health care licenses or approvals for health care services to be delivered.) Under a sole proprietorship, an owner can combine assets, using one checking account for business and personal purposes and one account for taxes owed on his or her tax returns. The sole proprietor, however, is also personally liable for all debts of the business. If a sole proprietor decides to share the responsibilities of the business with another person or party, the sole proprietorship will immediately and automatically be viewed legally as another entity, such as a partnership, regardless of the intent of the parties (Ballard, Mitchell-Stoddard, & Radney, 2011).

PARTNERSHIPS

There are a number of types of partnership entities, of which full discussion is beyond the scope of this chapter. In general, however, a partnership is the relationship existing between two or more persons who join together to carry on a trade or business. Each partner contributes money, property, labor, or skill, and expects to share in the profits and losses of the business. A partnership is created under the laws of the state where the business is to be carried out. A partnership must file annual IRS information returns to report income, deductions, gains, losses, and so on, from the operations, but it does not pay income tax. Instead, it "passes through" any profits or losses to its partners. Each party includes its share of the partnership's income or loss on its personal tax return (Ballard, Mitchell-Stoddard, & Radney, 2011).

Persons contemplating conducting business in any partnership-type relationship should consult counsel for advice on its formation and operation.

LIMITED LIABILITY COMPANY

A limited liability company (LLC) is a flexible business structure that blends characteristics of partnerships and corporations. LLCs provide greater protection for members to manage the business and shield themselves from personal liability for the debts and obligations of the business. LLCs are allowed by state statutes, which vary from state to state. LLCs are a popular choice because, similar to a corporation, owners have limited personal liability for the debts and actions of the LLC. Other aspects of the LLC operate more like a partnership, providing management flexibility and the benefit of pass-through taxation (Ballard, Mitchell-Stoddard, & Radney, 2011).

Owners of an LLC are called members. Generally, there is no maximum number of members, and most states also permit single-member LLCs, which have only one owner. Certain types of businesses, such as banks and insurance companies, cannot operate as LLCs. State filings are required to start an LLC, and most LLCs maintain a separate operating agreement. It is necessary to review the relevant state statute and federal tax regulations for starting a business with this structure (Ballard, Mitchell-Stoddard, & Radney, 2011).

FIDUCIARY DUTIES: DUTIES OF CARE AND LOYALTY

A fiduciary duty is a legal obligation to act in the best interests of another party. In corporate matters, an example of a fiduciary duty is that which exists between a corporation's board members and the corporation he or she serves. Fiduciary duties fall into two broad categories—the duty of loyalty and the duty of care (Ballard, Mitchell-Stoddard, & Radney, 2011).

Duty of Care

The duty of care is a standard of behavior that requires a board member to exercise the same reasonable care that an ordinary, prudent person would exercise in a like position under similar circumstances. Reasonable care has two elements: (1) the board must be acting in good faith for the benefit of the company and the board members must believe that the actions they are taking are in the best interests of the company, and (2) that the actions taken are in the best interests of the company based on a reasonable investigation of the options available. To exercise this duty of care, board members must attend meetings and must be fully informed about the activity of the organization in order to be able to make informed and independent decisions when voting (Ballard, Mitchell-Stoddard, & Radney, 2011).

Duty of Loyalty

The duty of loyalty is a standard that requires board members to act in good faith, be faithful to the company, and pursue the company's best interests. The duty of loyalty is the duty of constant and unqualified fidelity (Ballard, Mitchell-Stoddard, & Radney, 2011).

A breach of the duty of loyalty would be *self-dealing*, which means taking a corporate opportunity and using it to benefit oneself instead of the corporation. In order to help eliminate the problem of self-dealing, corporate directors are advised to provide full disclosure of any issues that could cause a potential conflict of interest. A conflict of interest is a situation that occurs when a person's individual interests in a matter are such that his or her ability to act fully on behalf of the corporation is in question. If a conflict of interest occurs, the board member should disclose the conflict and remove himself or herself from voting on the conflicted matter (Ballard, Mitchell-Stoddard, & Radney, 2011).

FAST FACTS in a NUTSHELL

A fiduciary duty is a legal obligation to act in the best interests of another party. A fiduciary duty exists between a corporation's board member and the corporation he or she serves. Fiduciary duties fall into two broad categories—the duty of loyalty and the duty of care.

SUMMARY

Corporate law includes the laws and regulations governing legal entities that may be formed to conduct business, and describes the attributes of the various structures. Nurses can benefit from knowledge of corporate and business law to better understand the operation of the organization they are affiliated with and to assist them in the event they desire to start their own business. Nurses should also understand the nature of a fiduciary duty, which is the legal obligation of a corporate board member to act in the best interests of the corporation he or she serves.

16

Hospital Corporate Liability

Diana C. Ballard

Historically, hospitals were charitable institutions, and because of this were given immunity from being sued for negligence under a doctrine known as "charitable immunity." This was a protective stance, so that these charitable institutions would be able to raise money and continue their capability to serve their communities. As health care developed as a business, this approach changed, and the doctrine of hospital corporate liability evolved (Ballard, Mitchell-Stoddard, & Radney, 2011).

In this chapter, you will learn:

1. The key areas of responsibility of hospital corporations
2. To identify the articulated duties owed by hospitals to patients

RESPONSIBILITY OF HOSPITAL CORPORATIONS

A key question has been whether a hospital is liable for the negligent acts of a physician or other practitioner who is not

137

an employee of the hospital. It is already known that hospitals or health care organizations can be held liable for the acts of their employees and agents under the theory of *Respondeat Superior.* Physicians, however, have traditionally been independent contractors and not subject to the same controls with respect to their work; therefore, under traditional legal theories, a hospital was not liable for their acts (Ballard, Mitchell-Stoddard, & Radney, 2011).

The prevailing theory now governing hospital corporate responsibility is the Doctrine of Corporate Liability, which seeks to impose liability on hospitals for the negligence of physicians and other health practitioners, particularly when these persons are not employees. This theory recognizes that patients generally do not have control over certain medical services they may receive from physicians who work at the hospital as independent contractors. Anesthesiologists, radiologists, and pathologists are often examples of such services provided to patients without a patient's input or control. Hospitals' medical staff generally approves policies of certain medical and professional practitioners. Furthermore, patients rely on the reputation of the hospital in choosing where to go for their health care needs and services. As a result, the courts have taken the position that a physician is acting under the authority of the hospital when that authority has not in reality been granted through a relationship such as employment. This is known as the theory of "ostensible agency" (Ballard, Mitchell-Stoddard, & Radney, 2011).

The Doctrine of Corporate Liability was first applied in the case of *Darling v. Charleston Community Hospital* (1965). The case was brought on behalf of a minor patient who was being treated for a leg injury. The case alleged negligent care on the part of the hospital that resulted in amputation of the patient's leg. In its defense, the hospital argued that it could not be held responsible since a hospital does not practice medicine and that the only duty it owed to its patients was limited to using reasonable care in selecting medical doctors for its staff. The court, in reaching its decision, drew on The Joint Commission standards, the hospital's own bylaws, and other documents in outlining the extent of the hospital's responsibility, and held that the hospital owed an independent duty of care to the patient (Ballard, Mitchell-Stoddard, & Radney, 2011).

====================*FAST FACTS in a NUTSHELL*

A hospital owes an independent duty of care to the patient.

DUTIES OWED TO PATIENTS

Subsequent cases continued to refine the concept of corporate negligence, delineating the sources of standards that a plaintiff could offer as to hospital negligence. Accordingly, the duties of the hospital have been identified as:

1. The duty to use reasonable care in the maintenance of safe and adequate facilities and equipment
2. The duty to select and retain only competent physicians
3. Duties to oversee all medical care
4. The duty to formulate, adopt, and enforce adequate rules to ensure quality care for the patients (Nathanson, 1993)

At least 33 states have adopted or recognized corporate liability, imposing these or similar duties upon their hospitals (Weinstock & Chopko, 2008).

SUMMARY

The traditional theory of *Respondeat Superior* imposes liability upon an employer for the acts of the employee. The Doctrine of Corporate Liability seeks to impose liability on hospitals for the negligence of physicians and other health practitioners, particularly in cases when these persons are not employees. At least 33 states have adopted or recognized corporate liability, imposing specific duties upon their hospitals.

17

Continuous Quality Improvement and Risk Management

Diana C. Ballard

Health care risk management consists of ensuring a safe environment and reducing risks to individuals and health care organizations, both areas in which nurses play a vital role. Nurses are essential participants in the design, development, and implementation of an organization's risk management program, and will benefit from knowing the basics of such a program and the resources needed for an effective plan (Miller, 2011).

In this chapter, you will learn:

1. The essential elements basic to a risk management program
2. High-risk areas for health care organizations and nurses
3. Methods to analyze risks and to implement changes that will reduce risk and promote quality improvement

THE RISK MANAGEMENT PROGRAM

An effective risk management program requires the constant application of several key elements:

- Integration into the operations of the health care organization
- Open lines of communication and data sharing
- Accountability of clinical leaders
- Authority of designated risk officer to implement and enforce the plan. (Miller, 2011)

A complete risk management program involves and engages a number of key individuals in the organization. This may include a patient safety officer, quality manager, human resource professionals, and more. Much of the structure is dependent on the size and resources of the organization. In some organizations, certain roles will have a designated manager, and in other organizations, individuals can serve in multiple roles. Whatever the structure of the organization and its resources, the keys to effective operation of the risk management program are collaboration, coordination, and communication among those responsible for these key processes and functions.

========================*FAST FACTS in a NUTSHELL*

Keys to the effective operation of a risk management program are collaboration, coordination, and communication among those responsible for key processes and functions.

RISK IDENTIFICATION

A key tool in identifying risks in an organization is reviewing and analyzing "occurrence" or "incident" reports. These reports provide an early warning system, intended to identify risk situations or adverse events. The reports can signal the start of an investigation and can result in corrective actions to avoid similar situations from recurring.

Today such events are more likely to be electronically recorded and reported. Whether done manually or electronically, the report is most effective when filed as close to the time of the incident being reported as possible, as the events will be fresh in the mind of the reporter, and the report is likely to contain the most accurate and complete description of events. The report should contain only the facts, as objectively presented as possible. Occurrence reports may be seen by others outside the organization at some point in the future, so including any extraneous or nonpertinent information in them should be avoided (Miller, 2011).

Electronic reporting systems do offer some advantages. Some electronic systems are Web based, allowing for contact through multiple facilities, with immediate e-mail notification to clinical managers and access by risk managers. If an event occurs that suggests or poses a significant danger or risk to others, then the reporter should advise the risk manager or administration immediately. The written report should be carried out; however, a dangerous situation should be addressed immediately in order to effect a timely response and avoid further harm (Miller, 2011).

Incident or occurrence reports are not tools to measure individual performance. In fact, use in this manner is more likely to have a negative effect, in that there may be a reluctance to file reports for fear of personal reprisal. The risk identification and occurrence reporting programs are based on self-reporting. Therefore, it is important to avoid using such reports as a basis for employee discipline (Miller, 2011).

Additional means of reporting events can include patient safety hotlines, e-mail notification systems, or direct person-to-person reports. Routine risk management rounding in all areas of the facility can also identify areas of risk. Other sources of information include routine review of medical record requests, results of patient surveys, and review of diagnostic codes upon discharge. Nurses are in a good position to identify risks in their work area and should welcome the opportunity to participate in rounds, surveys, or other risk management activities (Miller, 2011).

═══════════════════════════════*FAST FACTS in a NUTSHELL*

"Occurrence" or "incident" reports provide an early warning system that can identify risk situations or adverse events; thus they should be carefully reviewed and analyzed.

RESPONDING TO ADVERSE EVENTS

The scope of adverse events is broad, including any unintended or unfavorable event that involves a patient, whether or not it causes harm to the patient.

If a patient has been injured or has suffered ill effects, the nurse must first stabilize the patient and secure the necessary resources to help the patient and help transition the patient to the next level of care as needed. The nurse should activate the facility's chain of command in order to get whatever assistance is needed in the situation. This also enables senior administration to be aware and in a position to approve the deployment of resources and services as may be needed (Miller, 2011).

Beyond securing and providing the care needed for the patient, there are other steps that should be taken. The organization should have a policy in place whereby the patient's bill can be put on hold until it is determined what services may have been required due to the adverse event. Expenses necessitated by medical or hospital error should not be borne by the patient. In fact, Medicare may deny payment if the event is one of the "serious adverse events" that the Centers for Medicare and Medicaid Services (CMS) have determined are reasonably preventable (see discussion in Chapter 19). It is important to secure all evidence that may be relevant to the event. This may include medical equipment, devices, clinical records, or other items. The complete medical record should be secured and sequestered to ensure that the record as it existed at the time of the event is not altered (Miller, 2011).

ROOT CAUSE ANALYSIS AND SENTINEL EVENT DETERMINATION

A sentinel event as defined by The Joint Commission is an un-expected occurrence involving death, or serious physical or psychological injury, or the risk thereof. A root cause analysis is a problem-solving process used to determine the root cause or causes of an occurrence or event. Nurses may be asked to participate in a meeting to determine whether a sentinel event has occurred.

A root cause analysis can be employed to analyze either a sentinel event or an event that is not considered a sentinel event. In either case, an appropriate response includes the following:

- Conducting a timely, thorough, objective, and credible root cause analysis
- Developing an action plan designed to implement improvements in order to reduce risk or recurrence of the same or similar events
- Effectively implementing the improvements
- Monitoring the effectiveness of the improvements. (Miller, 2011)

FAST FACTS in a NUTSHELL

A root cause analysis is a problem-solving process used to determine the root cause or causes of an occurrence or event.

PEER REVIEW AND CONFIDENTIALITY

State laws vary, and depending on the laws of your state, the sentinel event and root cause analysis processes may be considered peer review and therefore kept confidential. Peer review, medical peer review, and performance improvement activities have been given confidential status in many states. This encourages a thorough and critical review of events by health care providers who would otherwise feel vulnerable if those proceedings could be made public. Nurses should be aware of the peer review and quality improvement policies in their facilities and should follow those policies so that the full benefit of the protective laws and the privacy of the records of such proceedings can be achieved (Miller, 2011).

REGULATORY REQUIREMENTS

Some states have statutes and regulations requiring notification of state authorities when an adverse event occurs. Currently, 26 states required some form of reporting of certain defined adverse events. In addition, other regulatory agencies may require notification in connection with specific events, such as the Food and Drug Administration if an event involves pharmaceutical or medical devices, or Medicare in cases in which a patient death occurred and restraints or seclusion was used within a specified time period (42 CFR §482.13 [g]). Again, the risk management, legal, or compliance departments are the sources of authority on these requirements, including the specific manner of filing the report, and nurses should be familiar with the relevant policies and seek advice from the appropriate department official (Miller, 2011).

INFORMING PATIENTS

Organizations have varying policies and procedures for disclosing information to patients or families with regard to any adverse occurrences. Any such disclosure should take place according to the policies and methods in place for such discussions. When the disclosure is made, the nurse should be prepared to provide whatever support is needed by the patient and family (Miller, 2011).

Opinion is divided on making apologies to patients when an adverse event has occurred. Some facilities, on advice of counsel, do not recommend this as they believe it does amount or may amount to an admission of wrongdoing. Others believe that a properly delivered and sincere apology is appropriate for the patient or family in such situations and can also contribute to reduced incidence of litigation. Some states have enacted so-called sorry laws, which prohibit an apology from being admissible as evidence in a civil action (Ballard, 2011).

Nurses should be familiar with the relevant organizational policy and should follow it precisely. Given the opportunity, nurses should participate in discussions leading to development of the organization's policy.

CARE FOR THE CAREGIVERS

Involvement in an adverse event can be distressing and even traumatic for the staff. When such a situation occurs, it is important for the staff to have the opportunity to communicate their feelings surrounding the event, and to receive the necessary emotional support. In a catastrophic event, a formal debriefing may be necessary to help facilitate the discussions and promote caregiver healing. These activities must be carried out in a secure and confidential environment (Miller, 2011).

SUMMARY

Health care risk management consists of ensuring a safe environment and reducing risks to individuals and to health care organizations. Nurses are essential participants in the design, development, and implementation of an organization's risk management program. Occurrence reports provide an early warning system to identify risk situations or adverse events, and should not be used as a tool to measure individual performance. Nurses should know their organizations' policies with regard to procedures employed in responding to adverse events, including peer review and quality improvement policies, so that the full benefit of protective laws and privacy of proceedings can be achieved. Some adverse events are distressing and traumatic for staff; accordingly, hospitals should have secure and confidential procedures in place to assist staff in dealing with such situations.

18

Corporate Compliance

Diana C. Ballard

Compliance is being in conformance with the requirements of laws, regulations, policies, procedures, and
conduct. The laws and regulations governing health care
compliance are numerous and complex. Compliance
requirements apply to numerous business and service
arrangements among and between hospitals, physicians,
freestanding surgery centers, skilled nursing facilities,
and other health care facilities and entities (Ballard,
2011).

The penalties for noncompliance can be severe. In
some cases the relevant laws are criminal statutes, and
penalties can include imprisonment. In both civil and
criminal cases, penalties can include significant monetary penalties and even exclusion from participation
in any governmental health program. The more knowledgeable health care professionals are with respect to
compliance requirements, the more likely the organization is to have a successful compliance program
(Ballard, 2011).

In this chapter, you will learn:

1. The concept of corporate compliance, including the framework of law and regulation that governs compliance
2. The key elements, benefits, and requirements of an effective corporate compliance program
3. The role of nurses with regard to corporate compliance, including the impact on nursing practice and responsibilities

ORIGINS OF CORPORATE COMPLIANCE

The federal government began focusing on health care fraud and abuse in the 1990s, owing to concerns over the amount of money that was being spent to support the Medicare program (Michael, 2003).

The Health Insurance Portability and Accountability Act (HIPAA) of 1996 established a national program to control health care fraud and abuse. This program is under the joint direction of the Attorney General and the Secretary of the Department of Health and Human Services (DHHS), acting through the Inspector General, and is designed to coordinate federal, state, and local law enforcement activities with respect to health care fraud and abuse (HIPAA of 1996, Public Law 104–191; the Balanced Budget Act [BBA] of 1997, Public Law 105–133).

Corporate compliance has as its legal basis the Federal Sentencing Guidelines that came into force in 1991 and imposed stiff penalties and sanctions for corporations convicted of wrongdoing.

> It is estimated that fraud, waste, and abuse make up between 3% and 10% of this country's $1-trillion annual health care expenditures. During the fiscal year 1997 alone, the Medicare program reported that $20.3 billion—11% of all Medicare fee-for-service payments— was due to fraud and abuse. (Fowler, 1999, p. 50)

The only mitigating factors that can significantly reduce sanctions and penalties for violations of compliance requirements are those associated with an effective program to prevent violations of law, to encourage self-reporting of violations, and to cooperate with authorities in investigations. Corporate Compliance Programs (CCPs) that include these elements can facilitate risk reduction in areas of civil and criminal liability (Fowler, 1999).

Compliance enforcement programs have produced results. In its Annual Performance Report for Fiscal Year 2008, the DHHS, Office of the Inspector General (OIG) reported that the return on investment measuring the efficiency of the OIG's health care oversight effort continued its trend of increasing returns and reached $17 for every dollar spent on enforcement efforts for the reporting period (Message from the Inspector General, 2008).

=== *FAST FACTS in a NUTSHELL*

An effective program to prevent violations of law, to encourage self-reporting of violations, and to cooperate with authorities in investigations is the only mitigating factor that can significantly reduce sanctions and penalties for violations of compliance requirements.

MEDICARE CONDITIONS OF PARTICIPATION (COP)

Organizations that participate as providers of services in the Medicare program must meet specific standards as set forth by the Centers for Medicare and Medicaid Services (CMS) in the Conditions of Participation (CoP). CoP are identified by the CMS as minimum health and safety standards that are the foundation for improving quality and protecting the health and safety of beneficiaries (CMS, n.d.). Organizations must know the CoP that are relevant to the type of services they provide.

The secretary of the DHHS may refuse to enter into an agreement or may terminate an agreement after determining that a hospital (or other provider or entity) fails to substantially meet this definition, thus removing a provider's eligibility to participate as a provider in the Medicare program (42 U.S.C. Section 1395x[e]).

OIG COMPLIANCE GUIDANCE FOR HOSPITALS

To assist in its antifraud and abuse efforts, the DHHS' OIG encourages health care facilities to develop corporate compliance programs, and publishes model guidance to assist in the structuring and effective performance of such programs. Guidance programs can be found on the OIG website (visit http://www.oig.hhs.gov/). OIG guidance documents are available for a number of organization and business types, including but not limited to:

- ambulance suppliers
- clinical laboratories
- DMEPOS (durable medical equipment, prosthetics, orthotics, and supplies) industry
- individual and small-group physician practices
- home health agencies
- hospices
- hospitals

The OIG prepares and publishes its "work plan" annually. The OIG work plan is an important tool for determining what priority areas their work will address for the upcoming year. Compliance departments use this as one of the sources of information that serves as a basis for the development of their organization's annual compliance work plan (Ballard, 2011).

==*FAST FACTS in a NUTSHELL*

The OIG work plan, published annually, is an important tool to use in developing an organization's own annual compliance work plan.

LEGAL FRAMEWORK: LAWS THAT FORM THE LEGAL BASIS FOR COMPLIANCE

The Civil False Claims Act

The Civil False Claims Act (FCA; 31 U.S.C. S3729–33) is the primary federal statute that defines how the government can determine whether a person may be held responsible or may have liability for making a false claim. To summarize, under the FCA, liability can be found if it is determined that a person knowingly presents, or causes to be presented, a false claim that is paid or approved, allowed, or claimed. For purposes of this statute, "knowing" means that a person has actual knowledge of the information, or acts in deliberate ignorance of the falsity or truth of the information, or acts in reckless disregard of the truth of the information. The FCA was amended in 1986 to expand the types of claims that could be prosecuted and to lower the level of proof necessary to recover payments (Smith, 1999). This changed the nature of medical billing and coding inaccuracies in that they can be a basis for exclusion in addition to heavy fines and penalties (Ballard, 2011).

The Antikickback Statute

The antikickback statute (42 U.S.C. s1320a–7b[b]) is a criminal statute that prohibits a person from "knowingly and willfully" giving or offering to give "remuneration" if that payment is intended to constitute an "inducement" that will influence the recipient to:

- "refer" an individual to a person for the furnishing of any item or service for which payment may be made, in whole or in part, under a federal health care program (a covered item or service)
- "purchase," "order," or "lease" any covered item or service
- "arrange for" the purchase, order, or lease of any covered item or service, or
- "recommend" the purchase, order, or lease of any covered item or service

The antikickback statute also prohibits the solicitation or receipt of remuneration for any of these purposes. The statute is very broad, and it is important to consult counsel when entering into relevant transactions to see whether the arrangement contemplated meets the legal requirements of any exception or safe harbor under the law that may exist (Ballard, 2011).

Stark II Act 42 U.S.C. 1395nn

According to CMS, Stark Law serves to curb overutilization of services, prevent limitations on a patient's choice of services based on financial considerations, and avoid restricting competition. The Stark Law, often referred to as the antireferral law, prohibits a physician from making a referral

- to a health care entity
- for the furnishing of a designated health service (DHS)
- for which payments may be made under Medicare or Medicaid, and
- if the physician or an immediate family member has a financial relationship with the entity

For Stark Law purposes, a financial relationship is defined broadly and includes almost any form of compensation arrangement, direct or indirect. DHSs are explicitly named and published by the current procedural terminology code annually. The DHS categories included in the list of codes are as follows:

- clinical laboratory services
- physical therapy services (including speech–language pathology services)
- occupational therapy services
- radiology and certain other imaging services
- radiation therapy services and supplies

Other categories may also be considered a DHS in addition to those listed, and counsel should be consulted when reviewing arrangements.

If a financial relationship as defined under Stark exists and patients are referred for a DHS, then the activity must either comply with an exception or the activity is illegal. Compensation arrangements that constitute an exception under Stark Law include, among other things, bona fide employment arrangements, rental of office space or equipment, and physician recruitment. To repeat, activities should be carefully analyzed by counsel fully informed of the specifics of the arrangement to ensure that the arrangement is structured as required in order to be in compliance with Stark. The Stark Law is one of the most complex laws in the health care arena (Ballard, 2011).

═══════════════════════════════*FAST FACTS in a NUTSHELL*

The Stark Law is often referred to as the antireferral law. Arrangements should be carefully analyzed by counsel in order to confirm that the arrangement is structured as required.

The Emergency Medical Treatment and Labor Act

The Emergency Medical Treatment and Labor Act (EMTALA) requires hospitals to provide appropriate medical screening to any person who comes to the hospital emergency department and requests treatment or an examination for a medical condition. The law arose from several high-profile reports of patients needing emergency care and treatment but who were not treated in hospital emergency rooms because they did not have insurance or could not afford to pay (Ballard, 2011).

Congress enacted EMTALA, which applies to any facility that participates in Medicare and has an emergency department, including military and Veterans Administration facilities (Assid, 2007). Virtually all hospitals in the United States participate in Medicare. EMTALA covers all persons treated at those hospitals, not just those who receive Medicare benefits. Under EMTALA rules, patients who go to a covered provider seeking care for an emergency condition must be given a medical screening examination (MSE). The purpose of the MSE is to determine whether or not an emergency medical condition exists or whether a patient is in active labor. The person carrying out the MSE must be properly trained and qualified to do the examination, and must be credentialed under the organization's bylaws and governing documents. Proper training under EMTALA means that the person has had specific training in conducting the MSE to determine whether or not an emergency medical condition exists. Triage does not constitute an MSE unless the nurse carrying out the triage has had specialized training to conduct the MSE and is specifically credentialed through the hospital's medical staff credentialing process. For pregnant patients, the practice of conducting triage in the emergency department and sending the patient to the hospital's labor and delivery suite for the MSE is acceptable (Ballard, 2011).

EMTALA does not prohibit asking patients about their method of payment for the emergency department visit (Assid, 2007). Federal law permits the obtaining of information in the routine registration process, but the MSE or stabilizing treatment cannot be delayed because such information is not available or obtaining of such information is under way. In addition, EMTALA does not permit such information to be obtained "under duress." For patients presenting at an emergency room, this becomes a crucial factor because the experience of going to or being in an emergency room can be stressful. Accordingly, many hospital emergency departments do not initiate inquiries into insurance coverage or payment arrangements at least until the MSE has been completed, including consideration of the patient's condition at the time. However, hospitals must take care that such inquiries do not result in any delay in screening, stabilization, or treatment obligations under EMTALA (Ballard, 2011).

═══════════════════════════*FAST FACTS in a NUTSHELL*

Hospitals must take care that inquiries into insurance coverage or payment arrangements do not result in any delay in screening, stabilization, or treatment obligations under EMTALA.

If the examination reveals an emergency condition or active labor, the hospital must stabilize the condition. If the hospital is incapable of providing the necessary treatment, it may transfer the patient after stabilization.

In a July 13, 2006, memo from the CMS, the agency clarified that a hospital has an EMTALA obligation at the time a person "presents" at a hospital's dedicated emergency room or on hospital property other than the emergency room and requests treatment or examination for an emergency medical condition. This memo resulted from reports of "parking" as a hospital's practice of preventing the transfer of patients from the emergency medical services stretcher to the hospital bed or stretcher (CMS, 2006).

Hospitals mistakenly believed that until they actually took responsibility for the patient, they were not obligated to provide care or accommodate the patient. CMS pointed out in the memo that such practices may be a violation of EMTALA and that the EMTALA obligation is triggered at the time the patient "presents," as discussed previously.

SUMMARY

Compliance is being in conformance with the requirements of laws, regulations, policies, procedures, and conduct. The HIPAA of 1996 established a national program to control health care fraud and abuse. The only mitigating factors that can significantly reduce penalties for violation of compliance requirements are those associated with an effective CCP. An effective program includes, among other things, monitoring to prevent violations of law, self-reporting of violations, and cooperation with authorities in investigations. Nurses should participate in compliance education programs and should be familiar with the procedures in place in their organizations to report issues or raise questions.

PART

VII

Disasters and Public Health Emergencies

19

Legal Framework and Response Coordination

Diana C. Ballard

Public health emergencies can emerge from a number of situations. As we have seen in recent years, they can be weather-related natural disasters such as was experienced in Hurricane Katrina in 2005; intentional acts of individuals or organizations, such as 9/11; disease incidence or threats such as the H1N1 pandemic of 2009; or technological disasters such as the one that occurred in Chernobyl in 1996, where systems failure led to a nuclear disaster.

Whatever the cause of the emergency, it is important to be aware of how the disaster is defined, what aspects of a disaster can help to describe its nature and scope, what a declaration of emergency is and how it is made, and what apparatuses exist for organization and management of the response.

In this chapter, you will learn:

1. The definition, causes, and common characteristics of a disaster or emergency situation
2. The process of and responses to a declaration of emergency
3. A select summary of the relevant framework of law, regulation, standards, and guidelines governing communication and response coordination

CAUSES OF DISASTERS AND PUBLIC HEALTH EMERGENCIES

Public health emergencies and disasters can come about as a result of disease outbreaks and pandemics, natural disasters, technological disasters, and intentional acts. The word *disaster* implies a sudden overwhelming and unforeseen event (Burnham & Rand, 2008).

There are characteristics that, although common to disasters, can vary greatly in nature and scope. For example, the word *disaster* signifies that the event that has occurred is such that it cannot be handled without outside help. Depending on the nature and extent of the event, this could mean that it is a homeowner who must obtain help from neighbors, a community that needs assistance from other communities, or a state that requires assistance from the federal government (Burnham & Rand, 2008).

════════════════════════════*FAST FACTS in a NUTSHELL*

An event that is described as a disaster indicates that a sudden overwhelming and unforeseen event has occurred and is such that it cannot be handled without outside help.

However, there is no standard measure to define the scope of a disaster. Depending on the nature of the event, it could be described by the scope of property damage or lives lost, among other things. Since there is such variation in the types of events possible, these aspects will vary depending on the nature of the disaster.

In trying to determine the nature and extent of a disaster, it will be necessary to obtain as much information as possible about what has happened, such as the cause of the event, what damage or loss of any type has been sustained, whether there is actual or risk of continuing activity or damage, and an estimate of how much and what type of assistance is needed. In this way, it will be possible to enact a response appropriate to the nature and scope of the disaster that has occurred.

REVIEW OF RELEVANT LEGAL FRAMEWORK

Robert T. Stafford Disaster Relief and Emergency Assistance Act (the Stafford Act) and the Federal Emergency Management Agency (FEMA)

With enactment of the Stafford Act in 1974 and the creation of FEMA in 1979, the federal government developed an apparatus to plan for and respond to natural disasters. Over time, the expansive language of the Stafford Act enabled presidents of the United States to rely on Stafford Act authority to respond to acts of terrorism in addition to disasters (Banks, 2011).

The Stafford Act authorizes the president to issue major disaster, emergency, and fire management declarations. The issuance of such a declaration enables federal agencies to provide assistance to state and local governments overwhelmed by catastrophes, and also enables the president to determine whether certain types of authorized assistance will be provided and the conditions under which the aid is distributed (McCarthy, 2007).

═══════════════════════════*FAST FACTS in a NUTSHELL*

The Stafford Act enables the president of the United States to issue emergency declarations that enable federal agencies to provide assistance to state and local governments that are overwhelmed by catastrophes.

The Stafford Act §401 requires that "all requests for a declaration by the president that a major disaster exists shall be made by the governor of the affected state." In this act, a state also includes the District of Columbia, Puerto Rico, the Virgin Islands, Guam, American Samoa, and the Commonwealth of the Northern Mariana Islands. The Marshall Islands and the Federated States of Micronesia are also eligible to request a declaration and receive assistance (42 U.S.C. 5121 et seq).

As set forth in the Stafford Act, a governor seeks a presidential declaration by submitting a written request to the president through the FEMA regional office. The governor must certify that the combined local, county, and state resources are insufficient and that the situation is beyond their recovery capabilities. If practical, as based on the nature of the emergency, state and federal officials will carry out a preliminary damage assessment (PDA) to arrive at an estimate of the scope and extent of the disaster and its impact on individual and public facilities. In usual circumstances, the governor's request follows the PDA; however, this can be modified in situations in which a severe catastrophic event requires immediate response. FEMA regional and national offices review the request and the submitted information and provide to the president an analysis of the situation with a recommended course of action. As part of the request, the governor must take appropriate action under state law and direct execution of the state's emergency plan (Centers for Disease Control and Prevention [CDC], n.d.).

On the basis of the governor's request, the president may declare that a major disaster or emergency exists, thus activating an array of federal programs to assist in the response and recovery effort. The determination of which programs are activated is based on the needs found during damage assessment and any subsequent information that may be discovered.

It should be noted, however, that when emergencies cross state and national borders, the federal government has independent authority. In addition, it should be noted that changes relating to the Stafford Act were made after Hurricane Katrina in order to improve response in major disasters. In any event, counsel experienced in such matters should be retained as needed to guide responses in disaster situations.

The Emergency Management Assistance Compact

The Emergency Management Assistance Compact (EMAC) was approved by Congress in 1996, and was adopted by all 50 states and 3 territories. EMAC's purpose is to facilitate interstate mutual aid and manage reimbursement and liability issues when a disaster arises (Allen & Harris, n.d.). Assistance under EMAC is triggered by a state declaration of emergency. A member state's request for assistance is routed to other member state(s) to fulfill the assistance request. Under EMAC, the "requesting state" pays costs to the "responding state," such as labor costs, material costs, and contractor costs. The federal government will reimburse costs paid to the "responding state" if the president has declared an emergency or disaster, and if the costs are eligible under the Stafford Act. States that are a party to a response under EMAC and their officers or employees are not liable for negligence while rendering aid. However, such persons may be liable for willful misconduct, gross negligence, or recklessness. See the discussion in Chapter 20 for more specific discussion of nurse licensing and liability issues under EMAC.

Homeland Security Act of 2002

The Homeland Security Act of 2002 required the Secretary of the Department of Homeland Security (DHS) to "consolidate existing Federal Government emergency response plans into a single, coordinated national response plan" (6 U.S.C. §312[6]). The act consolidated relevant agencies, including FEMA, into the department, and the Secretary was given authority and control over all of its officers and agencies. The act designates the DHS as the lead agency for coordinating disaster and emergency response and recovery assistance with state and local authorities (Banks, 2011).

DECLARATION OF EMERGENCY

The Constitution, under the 10th Amendment, grants enumerated powers to the federal government. These powers include, among others, the power to regulate interstate commerce, to provide for the national defense, and the power to tax and spend for public welfare. Powers not enumerated are "reserved" to states and include the primary "police power" function, which gives states the right to act in the interest of the health, safety, and general welfare of its residents. Every state and locality may exercise this fundamental police power to protect the public health and safety of its population.

Public health control powers are a subset of the police powers, and include:

- surveillance
- reporting

- epidemiological investigation
- vaccination (voluntary/involuntary)
- isolation (voluntary/involuntary)
- treatment (voluntary/involuntary)
- other social distancing measures
- evacuation
- powers over property (CDC, n.d.)

EXERCISE OF POLICE AND PUBLIC HEALTH CONTROL POWERS

Facts and circumstances must be present to enable governments, federal or state, to exercise the police powers as enumerated in the preceding section. Since the exercise of this authority can impinge upon the personal or property rights of citizens, they are permissible only in specific circumstances when necessary to protect the public. For example, absent specific emergency conditions that pose a serious threat to public health, there is no existing general authority for the federal government to mandate vaccinations to the public. However, the Department of Defense and the State Department can require vaccination of uniformed service personnel and certain other government employees.

As another example, evacuation may be ordered when necessary to remove people from a location that is under imminent threat. This can occur, for example, in the Florida Keys when a hurricane is approaching or in an area that is in the path of a dam that is about to collapse. When the threat has passed, the agency issuing the evacuation order can rescind it. As a note with regard to evacuation orders, after Hurricane Katrina, legislation was passed to require that people with disabilities or special needs be informed of an evacuation order.

================================*FAST FACTS in a NUTSHELL*

A state's police power gives it the right to take actions needed to protect the health and safety of its residents. Since the exercise of this authority can impinge upon the personal or property rights of citizens, they are permissible only in specific circumstances when necessary to protect the public.

In any situation in which conditions permit, it is important to seek advice of counsel in issuing such emergency orders to ensure that the circumstances have been properly reviewed and actions taken in conformance with applicable law.

SUMMARY

Public health emergencies and disasters can come about as a result of disease outbreaks and pandemics, natural disasters, technological disasters, and intentional acts. During a disaster or public health emergency, the governor of a state needing assistance may request Stafford Act support from the federal government. There is no standard measure to define the scope of a disaster; it can be described in scope of property damage or lives lost, among other things. The Homeland Security Act of 2002 designates the DHS as the lead agency for coordinating disaster and emergency response and recovery assistance with state and local authorities. Under specific circumstances, a state's police power gives it the right to take actions needed to protect the health and safety of its residents.

20

Roles of Organizations and Nurses in Disasters

Diana C. Ballard

Events in recent years have heightened awareness and have clarified the reality that emergencies and catastrophic situations can and do occur. For many reasons, nurses may be called to duty in situations that lack the control, order, and resources of the usual practice situation. As a result, issues arise with regard to licensure in other states and locales, liability under uncertain conditions, employment, and hospital and community preparedness.

In this chapter, you will learn:

1. The role and responsibility of nurses in emergency situations and the applicable standard of care
2. The mechanisms and laws that exist to manage issues of temporary licensure for practice across state lines
3. A hospital's responsibility to have a plan for response to and recovery from all hazards
4. Liability associated with professional practice in disaster situations

PRACTICE OF NURSING IN EMERGENCIES AND DISASTERS

Nursing practice within a state is based on licensure in that state, and is granted based upon review and determination that the nurse is properly qualified and meets all of that state's requirements for such licensure. State licensure may carry with it the responsibility to engage in emergency and disaster response activities if called upon by the governor or by his or her agent. Failure to do so can result in sanctions against the nurse or other licensed provider (Liang, 2008).

NURSING LICENSURE

In a disaster or public health emergency, coordination among professional licensing boards and state and federal governments is necessary to ensure that individuals affected by the catastrophic event receive necessary and appropriate care (Allen & Harris, n.d.). State laws vary on the question of visiting health care professionals' ability to practice during these times of need. Some states' provisions permit nurses licensed in another state to practice during a declared emergency, such as the example from the Nurse Practice Act of the State of Illinois below:

b) This Act does not prohibit the following:

(4) The practice of nursing by a nurse who holds an active license in another state when providing services to patients in Illinois during a bona fide emergency or in immediate preparation for or during interstate transit. (225 ILCS 65 Sec.50-15(b)(4).

================================*FAST FACTS in a NUTSHELL*

Nurse licensure is based on the laws of the state in which he or she practices. In order to ensure the availability of care to victims of a disaster, tools such as multistate compacts and expanded Nurse Practice Act provisions have been enacted to facilitate practice across state lines.

EMERGENCY MANAGEMENT ASSISTANCE COMPACT

Other states have become party to multistate compacts, such as the Emergency Management Assistance Compact (EMAC), which has been ratified by all 50 states. In activating the provisions of EMAC or other such compacts, it is necessary to review relevant state laws, as state statutes vary in the language and provisions applicable to their participation in the compact.

"EMAC is an organization ratified by Congress to facilitate interstate mutual aid and manage reimbursement and liability issues when a disaster arises" (Allen & Harris, p. 2). Each state adopts EMAC individually, and in general allows the receiving state to recognize permits, licenses, and certifications of those from other states who come to render assistance during the EMAC emergency. The receiving state may impose limits or conditions on one's professional practice, and thus it is important to know the legislation and provisions in your state of practice and in the state where assistance is to be provided. The licensure and immunity provisions in EMAC were designed to apply to state employees, not those in the private sector. However, some states have expanded EMAC coverage to include private citizens during the EMAC emergency (Allen & Harris, n.d.).

Nurse Licensure Compact

The Nurse Licensure Compact (NLC) was formed to provide for mutual recognition of registered nurses and licensed practical nurses in order to facilitate the practice of nursing across state lines without additional licensure, and has been enacted in 23 states (Grant, 2011). It requires a nurse to obtain a license in the state of permanent residence, and if that state is a party to the multistate compact, she or he may practice in other party states. Although it was designed to facilitate telenursing across state lines, it is beneficial in times of disaster (Allen & Harris, n.d.).

Uniform Emergency Volunteer Health Practitioners Act

The Uniform Emergency Volunteer Health Practitioners Act (UEVHPA) was enacted in 2006, initially in response to the hurricanes of 2005, in recognition of the difficulties with state laws that prevented health care professionals from quickly and legally providing much needed aid to states where great damage and hardship had occurred (Allen & Harris, n.d.). At least 14 states have enacted UEVHPA (American College of Surgeons [ACS], 2012). During a declared emergency, states enacting UEVHPA recognize the licensure of physicians, nurses, and health practitioners from other states if those professionals have registered with a qualified public or private registration system. This permits those professionals to enter the state and provide services without having to seek a license in the state where the emergency has been declared (ACS, 2012). UEVHPA is activated when an authorized state or local official issues an emergency declaration and it continues in duration until discontinued or changed by the host state.

It applies to all volunteer practitioners who provide health or other specified services (Allen & Harris, n.d.). Practitioners are limited to the scope of practice allowed by their license in their home state, or the scope of practice allowed in the host state, *whichever is narrower* (Allen & Harris, n.d.).

═══════════════════════════*FAST FACTS in a NUTSHELL*

UEVHPA permits health care professionals to volunteer their services and provide needed care during emergency situations. In states where UEVHPA has been adopted, practitioners are limited to the scope of practice allowed by their home state, or by the host state, *whichever is narrower.*

LIABILITY ISSUES DURING EMERGENCIES

"No emergency changes the basic standards of practice, code of ethics, competence, or values of the professional" (American Nurses Association [ANA], 2008, p. 6). Medical care and resources during emergencies will be provided to the best extent possible. Decision making during extreme conditions shifts ethical standards from a focus on the individual to a focus on the greatest good for the greatest number of individuals. Care rendered is related to what is "sufficient given the specific conditions at the time" (ANA, 2008, p. 10).

Under extreme conditions it is likely that errors will occur and subsequently malpractice may be alleged. State and federal laws provide protection from liability for acting in good faith during emergencies. Further, it is important to recognize that in extreme conditions there will be increased reliance on all of one's accumulated competence, as the usual range of colleagues, experts, or support services may not be available (ANA, 2008, p. 12).

Good Samaritan Laws

Each state has enacted Good Samaritan laws to encourage health professionals to stop and render assistance at the scene of an accident or disaster (Karno, 2011). These laws vary greatly from state to state, and in general provide immunity from liability for negligent acts or omissions when rendering care in an accident, emergency, or under other specified circumstances. State laws typically condition the immunity on the basis that the service rendered was done in good faith and without fee (Karno, 2011).

================*FAST FACTS in a NUTSHELL*

It should be noted that in extreme conditions there will be increased reliance on all of one's accumulated competence, as the usual range of colleagues, experts, or support services may not be available.

HOSPITAL EMERGENCY OPERATIONS PLAN

Hospitals are required to have an emergency operations plan (EOP), which describes how a facility will respond to and recover from all hazards. It is important that nurses be involved in planning and preparing for community emergencies. The Joint Commission's emergency management standards for hospitals, critical access hospitals, and long-term care programs reflect an "all hazards" approach to emergency preparedness. This permits a flexible approach to emergencies as needed, based on the nature of the particular situation (ANA, 2008). The response is tailored, based on six critical areas of emergency management. It is inclusive of the six critical elements within The Joint Commission's Emergency Management Standards:

- communications
- resources and assets
- safety and security
- staff responsibilities
- utilities management
- patient clinical and support activities (ANA, 2008, p. 8)

The "all hazards" approach allows the ability to respond to a range of emergencies varying in scale, duration, and cause. The EOP addresses response procedures, capabilities, and procedures when the hospital cannot be supported by the community, recovery strategies, initiating and terminating response and recovery phases, activating authority, and identifying alternate sites for care, treatment, and services.

With regard to hospital operations during a time of emergency, it is important to note that the Emergency Medical Treatment and Active Labor Act imposes two principal obligations on hospitals participating in Medicare: (1) they must screen all individuals in the emergency room to determine whether or not an emergency condition exists, and (2) they must stabilize individuals before transferring or discharging. The Secretary of the Department of Health and Human Services can waive this requirement after declaring a public health emergency.

EMPLOYMENT AND RELEASE FROM WORK

The Uniformed Services Employment and Reemployment Rights Act of 1994 (USERRA) prohibits discrimination with regard to employment against persons on the basis of membership, application for service, or obligation for services in the armed forces. Some states have enacted laws patterned after USERRA. The Bioterrorism Preparedness and Response

Act extended USERRA's protections to certain federal emergency workers who may be sent to assist with national disasters. This includes employees who perform as intermittent disaster response appointees upon activation of the National Disaster Medical System, even if they are not members of the uniformed services (Fisher & Phillips, 2006).

USERRA restricts the treatment of employees who perform services protected by the statute. It provides three major categories of employer obligations:

- A person cannot be denied initial employment, reemployment, retention, promotion, or any benefit on the basis of his or her membership, application for service, or obligation for service in the armed forces
- Employers are required to provide eligible employees with up to 5 years of unpaid leave during the life of their employment; throughout this period, the employee's seniority, health care, and pension benefits must be maintained
- Returning service members have a virtually unfettered right to reemployment by their pre-service employers upon timely application for return to work (Fisher & Phillips, 2006).

To be eligible for protection under USERRA, the individual must hold a civilian job, provide advance written notice to the employer, report status to the employer on a reasonable time frame, and meet length of service requirements.

SUMMARY

In catastrophic situations, nurses may find themselves practicing in environments that lack control, order, and resources. Ethical standards change from a focus on the individual to a focus on the greatest good for the greatest number.

In order to facilitate practice across state lines in rendering care to those in need, multistate compacts and expanded practice acts have been enacted. Liability concerns are addressed in protective laws such as EMAC and Good Samaritan laws. Hospitals are required to have an EOP to guide actions during disasters. Nurses should participate in the development of such plans and should be familiar with the relevant laws as outlined in this chapter.

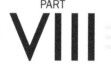

PART

VIII

Resolving Disputes

21

Anatomy of a Trial

Paula DiMeo Grant

In Part VIII: Resolving Disputes, trial procedure and alternative methods to resolve disputes such as negotiation, mediation, and arbitration will be covered. The American system of jurisprudence consists of civil and criminal courts on the state and federal levels. There are statutes of limitations as to when a case can be brought, with few exceptions. In a civil action, the injured party is called the plaintiff and the party sued is called the defendant (Plaintiff v. Defendant). In criminal actions, the party bringing the action is the government or the people against the person who allegedly committed the crime, the defendant (The People v. Defendant).

In this chapter, you will learn to:

1. Identify the steps in a civil trial
2. Describe the discovery process
3. Specify deposition tips

This chapter will primarily focus on the process of a civil trial.

CIVIL TRIAL PROCEEDINGS

Pretrial Phase: Civil Actions

The pretrial phase begins with a careful analysis, by competent counsel, of the facts of the case and the law as it applies to the facts. A review of the statute of limitations in addition to the four elements of a negligence claim, as previously discussed in Chapter 4, will be made. Statute of limitations is the time frame in which a case can be brought. Generally, a medical malpractice action must be brought within a relatively short period of time (1–3 years) from when the claim arose (when the legal duty was breached) or when the injuries became known to the plaintiff. This time frame varies from state to state. The exceptions to bringing an action within this time frame pertain to minors and/or individuals lacking the capacity to bring a cause of action. In those cases, the statute of limitations is extended.

The attorney may engage the services of an expert nurse or expert physician witness to determine whether there is a valid claim of medical malpractice. In some jurisdictions, medical malpractice certificates of merit are required from physicians, indicating that the case is legitimate or has merit. The information required varies from state to state, and not all states require a certificate of merit prior to filing a malpractice claim.

=================================*FAST FACTS in a NUTSHELL*

Statute of limitations is the time frame within which a lawsuit can be brought.

Plaintiff v. Defendant: Filing the Complaint

A lawsuit begins with the plaintiff filing a complaint alleging malpractice against the defendant in the appropriate court of law. A complaint is a legal document in the form of a statement of allegations, referred to as a pleading. It names the parties to the actions and it lists the allegations one by one of the wrongdoing in counts. Subsequently, the defendant is served the complaint. The defendant is given a certain period of time to respond to the complaint. If the defendant fails to answer the complaint within the prescribed period of time, as short as 20 days in some jurisdictions, a default judgment against the defendant may take place (Grant & Reardon, 2011).

Depending upon the circumstances, lawsuits may be instituted in state or federal courts (Figure 21.1). A court will have no authority to hear the case unless it has jurisdiction over the person or property involved in the matter. In the event that a nurse is named as a defendant in a medical malpractice case, it is imperative to notify his or her malpractice insurance carrier and/or a competent attorney as soon as practicable.

FAST FACTS in a NUTSHELL

A civil lawsuit begins with a plaintiff filing a "complaint" in a court of law against a defendant; the complaint alleges wrongdoing.

Discovery Process

An important part of the pretrial phase of a lawsuit is the discovery process. This process allows the parties to learn the details regarding the case. It also provides a formal mechanism for the parties to exchange information regarding evidence to be presented and witnesses that will be called to testify at trial. Discovery helps to define and clarify the issues presented. It is accomplished through the use of

THE COURT SYSTEM

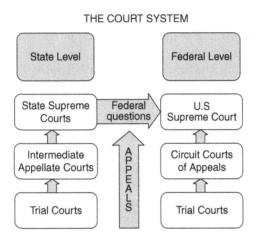

FIGURE 21.1   The court system.

interrogatories and/or depositions. There are rules of civil procedure pertaining to the discovery process that are adhered to by the courts.

Interrogatories

Interrogatories are series of questions relating to the lawsuit served upon the parties from the opposing sides. They are answered in writing and under oath. Interrogatories provide the parties with important information in preparation for depositions and trial. Requests for the production of documents may also be used to provide additional evidence or to clarify a question at issue. They may consist of certain records, documents, and tangible objects and are considered evidence. Interrogatories are to be answered within a specific time frame.

Depositions

A deposition is out-of-court testimony that is conducted by opposing counsel of witnesses or parties under oath and recorded by a court reporter or videotaped. Depositions allow the parties to learn the facts and issues of the case in a face-to-face setting. Testimony at a deposition can also be used to impeach or discredit a witness for inconsistent statements made at trial. Depositions provide a useful mechanism for discovery and preparation for settlement before trial or for trial (Grant & Reardon, 2011). If you are an expert witness in a case, you may be summoned to give a deposition.

══════════════════════════════*FAST FACTS in a NUTSHELL*

An important aspect of the pretrial phase is the discovery process. This process allows the parties to learn the details of the case through the mechanisms of interrogatories and depositions.

Deposition Tips

The following are tips for deposition preparation:

1. Preparation is the key.
2. Do a thorough review of all pertinent documents.
3. Be familiar with the deposition process.
4. Be sure to understand the question.
5. Answer *only* the questions asked.
6. You may ask to repeat the question if you do not understand it.
7. Answer the questions as succinctly as possible.
8. Be courteous.
9. Speak clearly.
10. Tell the truth. (Grant & Reardon, 2011)

If called to give a deposition, you will be prepared by the attorney representing you or the attorney who hired you as an expert witness.

Motions

Motions are requests made by either party to the judge for a legal ruling on a matter. Motions may only be made for legitimate reasons such as a motion to compel discovery, or a motion to dismiss a case because the case lacks a sound basis to go forward. There are also motions made for summary judgment if one party believes that there is no genuine issue of material facts that a jury needs to consider. The following case illustrates a motion for summary judgment.

CASE EXAMPLE

Hoard v. Roper Hospital, Inc., et al. (S.C. 2010)

Issue: Whether or not it was proper to reverse a summary judgment motion granted by the Lower Court to defendant radiologist.

SUMMARY OF FACTS: This tragic case involved a newborn who suffered from brain damage and paralysis as a result of alleged negligence of four defendants following the insertion of an umbilical vein catheter (UVC), which apparently was malpositioned and caused injuries. All defendants, except the radiologist, entered into a settlement agreement with the plaintiff.

The radiologist's motion for summary judgment was based on the fact that his alleged failures did not cause the catastrophic outcome. Thus, the radiologist argued that without the requisite element of causation, there could not be medical negligence. The attorneys for the radiologist further argued that the treating physician had reviewed the X-rays himself and made an independent decision not to reposition the UVC. Therefore, culpability, if any, simply rested with the treating physician.

COURT'S DECISIONS: The Lower Court agreed and granted the defendant radiologist's motion for summary judgment. The case was appealed to an intermediate court (the next highest court), which reversed the decision of the trial court. Upon appeal to the Supreme Court of South Carolina, the summary judgment in favor of the radiologist was reinstated (Brenner & Bal, 2010).

Pretrial Settlement

Following completion of the discovery process, parties may enter into settlement negotiations or attend mediation to facilitate settlement. Most courts require pretrial conferences to encourage settlement, and many cases do settle prior to trial. When the pretrial phase has been completed, if the case has not been dismissed or settled, it is ready for trial.

Trial Phase

Jury Selection

The trial phase begins with jury selection. Prospective jurors are screened to prevent bias on the jury by a process called *voir dire*. A series of questions will be asked to prospective jurors by the judge or attorney to assist in the jury selection process so that only impartial jurors are chosen. In some instances, juries may be given a questionnaire to complete (Grant & Reardon, 2011).

Burden of Proof

The plaintiff has the burden of proof, by a preponderance of the evidence, to prove all the allegations as set forth in the complaint, and in some cases there may be a higher standard to prove the allegations by clear and convincing evidence. Generally, in a medical malpractice action the standard to prove the allegations is by a preponderance of the evidence.

Opening Statements

After the jury has been selected, the trial begins with the attorneys for the parties making an opening statement. The purpose of the opening statement is to tell the jury what the case is about and how counsel plans to present evidence and testimony. The plaintiff's counsel will present first, followed by the defendant's counsel. During opening statements, the attorneys can be creative in their presentations to capture the jury's attention and present their case in the most favorable light to their client. The jury, however, is instructed not to consider the opening statement evidence (Grant & Reardon, 2011).

Presentation of Evidence

Generally, evidence in the form of testimony from witnesses and parties will be admissible in a court of law. Also included is documentary evidence in the form of written reports and the like that tend to prove the alleged facts. Hearsay evidence is usually not admissible in a court of law. Hearsay is an out-of-court statement used to prove the truth of the matter asserted. Admissible evidence is governed by the rules of evidence, which are strictly adhered to.

Evidence is presented by the attorneys for plaintiff and defendant by:

(a) Direct examination of witnesses and parties by "friendly" counsel
(b) Cross examination of witnesses and parties by "opposing" counsel
(c) Presentation of expert witnesses by the parties
  • qualifying the expert
  • presentation of the expert opinion (See Chapter 5 titled "Proving Malpractice: The Expert Nurse Witness").

At the close of the presentation of evidence of the plaintiff's case, the defendant may make a motion for a directed verdict by arguing that the plaintiff did not prove all the allegations by a preponderance of the evidence and therefore the defendant shall prevail.

Closing Arguments

Closing arguments provide an opportunity for counsel to go to the jury and give a summary of the case. Plaintiff's counsel wants the jury to believe that the burden of proof was met and that the jury should return the verdict in favor of his or her client. The defendant's counsel will take the opposite view. It is a time when counsel can highlight the case in a manner to keep the jury interested. During closing arguments, the art of persuasion is at play.

Jury Instructions: Jury Deliberations and Verdict

Following closing arguments, by counsel for the plaintiff and defendant, jury instructions are given to the jury by the judge. The judge reviews the rules of the court with the jury and also discusses what exhibits, if any, the jury is allowed to take into the jury room. A jury foreman is selected by the jury and announces the verdict at the end of deliberations. At times, a jury verdict form is used to assist the jurors with the application of the law to the facts of the case. The length of time the jury deliberates is determined by the jurors. Generally, the more complicated the case, the longer the deliberations. Depending upon the case, jurors may be sequestered during deliberations.

Posttrial Phase

Following the verdict, posttrial motions and appeals may be filed for a variety of reasons. For example, if the plaintiff was awarded a large monetary award, the defendant may file a motion to reduce the amount of money. The losing party may file an appeal to a higher court for review. Specific rules of law govern appeals.

SUMMARY

It is important for nurses to understand court proceedings to effectively participate in the legal process. A civil lawsuit begins with the plaintiff filing a complaint in the appropriate court of law that names the parties to the action and the allegations of wrongdoing. The statute of limitations provides for the time frame within which these actions can be brought. The standard for proving civil cases is by preponderance of evidence, or by clear and convincing evidence. As trials are costly and time consuming, alternative dispute methods are employed to reduce the number of trials necessary to resolve disputes.

22

Alternative Dispute Resolution

Paula DiMeo Grant

Alternative dispute resolution (ADR) is comprised of methods to resolve disputes, in most situations, outside the courthouse. Litigation can be costly and very time consuming. ADR provides mechanisms to reach amicable agreements and also preserve relationships. Those methods include negotiation, mediation, and arbitration. This chapter will describe those mechanisms and will discuss the role of the mediator in the mediation process. Bioethical mediation in health care settings will also be explored.

In this chapter, you will learn to:

1. Describe three dispute resolution methods
2. Identify the advantages of alternative dispute resolution (ADR)
3. Discuss The Joint Commission's conflict management standard
4. Discuss bioethical mediation

DISPUTE RESOLUTION METHODS

Negotiation

Negotiation is defined as a process between or among parties making offers of settlement by one party and accepted by another. It is a give-and-take process, and depending upon the complexity of the problem, it may be lengthy. Negotiation also requires good communication skills, and nurses have been trained in communication. Although nurses may not realize it, they negotiate in various ways to deliver optimum nursing care to their patients. Take, for example, workplace settings in which nurses negotiate with physicians and other staff members, vendors, family members, and patients themselves during the course of the workday.

It has been noted that negotiation with the following four basic points in mind will improve negotiating skills and lead to more productive outcomes.

Four Basic Points of Negotiation

1. People: Separate the people from the problem.
2. Interests: Focus on the interests and not on the positions.
3. Options: Generate a variety of options or possibilities before deciding what to do.
4. Objectivity: Insist that the result be based on some objective standard. (Fisher & Ury, 1981)

═══════════════════════════*FAST FACTS in a NUTSHELL*

Negotiation is defined as a process between or among parties making offers of settlement by one party and accepted by another. Nurses negotiate in various ways to deliver optimum patient care.

It is a known fact that some people are better negotiators than others. The more you negotiate, the more you gain confidence, and the better a negotiator you become. It is important that one be prepared for negotiation by knowing one's needs, setting goals, recognizing all issues, identifying the options available, and knowing what the other party wants. One must also bargain in good faith. Not all negotiations have a favorable outcome, even for the most seasoned negotiators. However, if negotiations fail, there are other ways to resolve matters that are effective and efficient and that can promote and maintain good relationships. Those methods include arbitration and mediation (Boulay & Grant, 2011).

Arbitration

Arbitration is a dispute resolution process whereby the parties agree in advance to abide by the decision of an arbitrator. Collective bargaining agreements contain arbitration clauses to resolve disputes. Arbitration is a process similar to that of a trial, but not as formal. The same rules of evidence that apply in court proceedings do not apply in arbitration proceedings. Nevertheless, arbitration allows for a hearing of the matter with both parties having an opportunity to be heard and to present their case. Decisions by arbitrators are usually upheld unless the arbitrator acted in an arbitrary and capricious manner when making the decision.

═══════════════════*FAST FACTS in a NUTSHELL*

Arbitration is a dispute resolution process whereby an arbitrator makes a decision following a hearing. Arbitration proceedings allow the parties to present their case before an arbitrator.

Mediation

Mediation is also known as facilitated negotiation; the facilitator is the mediator. A mediator is a neutral third party trained to assist the parties in the resolution of the dispute. The concept of mediation is one of voluntariness and empowerment of the parties. The goal of mediation is to reach an amicable agreement between the parties, an agreement that is fashioned by the parties. Unlike litigation, mediation is cost effective and usually confidential. In recent years, the process of mediation is being utilized in health care settings to resolve disputes.

Mediation Process: Six Stages

The following six stages describe the mediation process:

1. Mediator's Opening Statement

Introduction of the parties takes place during the opening statement. The mediator sets the rules for the session and describes the mediation process. There is also a question-and-answer session.

2. Case Presentation

The parties and/or counsel present their cases to the mediator in a group setting. This should be done without interruption. The mediator may take notes or ask questions for clarification purposes.

3. Issue Development and Discussion

The mediator organizes the issues, facilitates discussion, and identifies the common threads. The mediator also helps the parties to understand the issues that divide them.

4. Brainstorming

The mediator assists the parties in generating options or brainstorming for resolution. The mediator may meet with the parties individually or as a group during the brainstorming session.

5. Evaluation of Options

The options generated in the brainstorming stage are evaluated by the parties with the assistance of the mediator. It is here that options are accepted, rejected, or modified by the parties in working toward an acceptable agreement. This task is accomplished in individual and/or group sessions.

6. Agreement

The goal of mediation is to produce an agreement between the parties with terms and conditions outlined to resolve the dispute. In the event that an agreement is not reached at the end of the session, it may be necessary to conduct more than one mediation session. If an agreement is reached, it should be in writing and signed by the parties (Boulay & Grant, 2011).

The Role of the Mediator

A mediator is a facilitator, negotiator, and problem solver. Unlike a judge or an arbitrator, a mediator does not render decisions, but rather facilitates the discussion between the parties. The key factors in selecting a mediator are experience, background, knowledge, training, and areas of expertise. In general, there are no licensing requirements for mediators. There are, however, specialized courses sponsored by colleges, universities, and organizations. And in some instances, there are court-based programs especially designed for attorneys.

Mediators have no ownership of the dispute. Throughout the process, the mediator draws upon his or her background and experiences to problem solve, especially when an impasse occurs. The mediator does not decide who is right or wrong, and remains unbiased. The mediator plays a vital role in the process of mediation. The mediator will choose the method to mediate that suits his or her style and the case at hand (Boulay & Grant, 2011).

Characteristics of Effective Mediators

1. Neutrality
2. Understanding
3. Patience
4. Good listening skills
5. Good communication skills
6. Flexibility
7. Good judgment
8. Trustworthiness
9. Respect for others
10. Creativity

═══════════════════════════════*FAST FACTS in a NUTSHELL*

Mediation is facilitated negotiation with the mediator as the facilitator. The concept of mediation is one of voluntariness and empowerment of the parties.

Ethical Considerations in Mediation

Mediators, like other professionals, are bound by a code of ethics for mediators. They must adhere to the tenets of the code when accepting cases for mediation and during the process of mediation. Mediators must remain cognizant of conflicts of interest, impartiality, confidentiality, and the quality of the mediation process itself (*Dispute Resolution Magazine*, 2006).

Mediation Advantages

The advantages of mediation continue to be the efficacy of the process as it minimizes expense and oftentimes expedites resolution. Furthermore, the parties control the outcome by deciding their own remedies for settlement. Mediation is known to have positive effects on relationships by reducing bitterness and hostility. The process is becoming more popular in resolving health care disputes.

Bioethical Mediation

Bioethics takes into account the broad ranges of issues and ethical dilemmas in medicine and health care, which may include research, public health, end-of-life issues, and palliative care, as well as health care disparities (National Institutes of Health, 2012). Philosophers, health care providers, and theologians have contributed to its body of knowledge. Legal precedents in this area have also been established by the courts of this country in right-to-life cases. Additionally, legislation on the state and national levels has also played a significant role in the field of bioethics.

It is common for conflict to arise in health care settings regarding bioethical situations. Bioethical mediation has been implemented to assist in the resolution of ethical dilemmas. The process assists families, nursing, and medical staff members in making difficult end-of-life decisions in a dignified and responsible manner as illustrated by the following case study in bioethics mediation (Boulay & Grant, 2011). Ethical principles, as previously discussed, provide a framework and are utilized when resolving ethical dilemmas.

CASE STUDY

Bioethical Mediation

SUMMARY OF FACTS: Joseph was in the intensive care unit on life support. The prognosis for his recovery was grim, but there was the possibility that final surgery might save him. The likelihood of success was not great, considering Joseph's frail condition.

Victoria, his wife of 50 years, wanted the surgery; John, his son, who held a durable power of attorney over medical decisions, did not want the surgery. No one knew how long Joseph would live, and the hospital was concerned about the use of an expensive, scarce (sic) hospital bed. Joseph had instructed that no extraordinary means be used to prolong his life. A conflict evolved between the hospital, Victoria, and John over Joseph's future care. The hospital staff called a bioethics mediator to intervene, and the mediator consulted with the medical team and the nursing staff to better understand the medical situation. She asked the entire group who would be the most appropriate to represent the hospital and medical team. The medical resident and nurse agreed to participate.

The mediator met with Victoria and John, who were in a nearby waiting area close to Joseph's room. She sat down with them and explained that she was retained by the hospital in situations like this to help people find common ground. She briefly explained the process choice to Victoria and John. They agreed to participate in mediation.

THE MEDIATION PROCESS BEGINS: Victoria began by describing her long marriage to Joseph and her inability to accept his death. Her story was moving and tearful. The mediator gently summarized Victoria's story, creating an empathic connection with her. John spoke next about his love for his father, and his responsibility to carry out his father's wishes under the power of attorney. He hated the responsibility thrust on him and the fact that his obligation to his father conflicted deeply with his own needs and his mother's desires. Again, the mediator summarized John's perspective.

The mediator asked the resident and the nurse to give a summary of the medical situation. The mediator asked for clarification and simplification so Victoria and John could fully understand Joseph's condition. Victoria and John were invited to ask questions to clarify anything they did not understand.

ISSUE IDENTIFICATION: When everyone was satisfied that his or her stories had been told and heard, the mediator asked Victoria and John to identify the interests they needed satisfied to resolve the conflict. As the mediator assisted them in articulating their personal interests, everyone realized that John and Victoria were really aligned. The hospital's interests were expressed clearly by the resident and the nurse. First and foremost was Joseph's care.

OUTCOME: After further discussion, the tearful decision was made to remove Joseph from life support and provide him comfort and palliative care. Joseph passed on later that night (Noll, 2004, p. 1).

Bioethical Mediation Summary

This mediation example took place in a group or joint session with all parties present at all times. In this setting, the mother and son were able to articulate their stories and express their feelings in an open manner with all participants present. There was no animosity between mother and son as they discussed their mutual love for a husband and a parent, mutual love being a common thread. In addition, they were also able to hear the medical resident and nurse describe the medical condition of their loved one and that his care was paramount. This information brought some comfort to the family during this extremely difficult time. The ethical principles of autonomy and beneficence were also taken into consideration. The mediator was skillful in connecting with all the parties and able to summarize the various perspectives. The mediator showed a deep concern for the parties as well as a deep understanding of the issues at hand. The skills of active listening and good communication were also employed effectively in this example of mediation (Boulay & Grant, 2011).

Mediation in Other Health Care Settings

Medicare Mediation Program

The Centers for Medicare and Medicaid Services (CMS) implemented a mediation program nationwide. The program is designed to address complaints that do not include significant quality-of-care issues. It has been reported that 80% of beneficiary complaints are related to misunderstandings, poor communication, or patients' perception of care received (IPRO & CMS, 2003). Mediation provides a forum to address these concerns in a professional manner and in a confidential setting that empowers the participants to fashion their own remedies, unlike litigation. It has been reported that patients and physicians who participated in the pilot study reported satisfaction with the outcome.

Rush Model of Mediation

In 1995, Rush University Medical Center in Chicago instituted a successful mediation program that has become known as the "Rush Model" to resolve medical malpractice cases. A panel of experienced attorneys representing plaintiffs and defendants form the key element to this model of mediation. This program has proved successful in encouraging mediation instead of litigation for resolution of these matters (Blatt, Brown & Lerac, 2009).

Elder Mediation Programs

Elder mediation offers an opportunity for creative problem solving in the areas of probate, guardianship, and family caregiving, thus avoiding costly and time-consuming litigation. The state of North Carolina has implemented such a program (Curcio, 2009).

The Joint Commission's Conflict Management Standard

In 2009 The Joint Commission issued a "conflict management standard" to manage conflict in health care settings. The standard calls for the expanded use of mediation to resolve disputes as well as the development of a code of conduct that defines behaviors that are acceptable and unacceptable. It also calls for the development and implementation of a process to manage unacceptable behaviors. The standard also states that the governing body is ultimately responsible for the safety and quality of patient care that it provides (Bovio, 2009).

SUMMARY

Alternative Dispute Resolution offers efficient and effective methods of dispute resolution other than litigation. Negotiation and mediation enable the parties to decide their own remedies to settle disputes. Mediation uses a trained mediator to facilitate the process. Arbitration, on the other hand, is a dispute resolution tool whereby an arbitrator makes a decision after a hearing. Arbitration offers an alternative that is both less expensive and time consuming than litigation. There has been an increased use of these methods to resolve disputes in the health care arena, which has been quite successful. The trend is expected to continue.

References

Age Discrimination in Employment Act, 29 U.S.C. § 621 *et seq.*

Aging With Dignity. (n.d.). Retrieved from http://www.agingwith dignity.org

Allen, D. C., & Harris, S. F. (n.d.). *Licensure issues in the event of a disaster or emergency.* Retrieved from American Health Lawyers Association (AHLA) website: http://www.healthlawyers.org/ Members/PracticeGroups/THAMC/EmergencyPreparedness Toolkit/Documents/IX_Licensure/B_LicensureIssues DuringDisasterEmergency.pdf

American Arbitration Association, American Bar Association's Section of Dispute Resolution, & Association for Conflict Resolution. (2006). The model standards of conduct for mediators: September 2005. *Dispute Resolution Magazine,* 33–38.

American College of Surgeons. (2012, March 20). *Uniform Emergency Volunteer Health Practitioners Act (UEVHPA).* Retrieved from http://www.facs.org/ahp/uevhpa.html

American Nurses Association. (2001). *Bill of rights for registered nurses.* Washington, DC: Author.

American Nurses Association. (2001). *Code of ethics with interpretive statements.* Washington, DC: Author.

American Nurses Association. (2002, June 24). *Registered nurses' rights and responsibilities related to work release during a disaster.* Retrieved from http://nursingworld.org/workreleaseps

American Nurses Association. (2008, March). *Adapting standards of care under extreme conditions: Guidance for professionals during disasters, pandemics, and other extreme emergencies.* Retrieved from http://www.a2p2.com/mep-p/ethics/Adapting_Care_Guidance.pdf

Americans With Disabilities Act, 42 U.S.C. § 1201 *et seq.*

Assid, P. A. (2007). Emergency medical treatment and active labor act: What you need to know. *Journal of Emergency Nursing, 33*(4), 324–326.

Balanced Budget Act of 1997, Pub. L No. 105–133.

Ballard, D. (2011). Corporate compliance. In P. D. Grant & D. C. Ballard (Eds.), *Law for nurse leaders* (pp. 67–104). New York, NY: Springer Publishing Company.

Ballard, D., Mitchell-Stoddard, M., & Radney, L. (2011). Corporate law. In P. D. Grant & D. C. Ballard (Eds.), *Law for nurse leaders* (pp. 45–66). New York, NY: Springer Publishing Company.

Banks, W. C. (2011, February). *The legal landscape for emergency management in the United States.* Retrieved from www.Newamerica.net website: http://security.newamerica.net/sites/newamerica.net/files/policydocs/Banks_Legal_Landscape.pdf

Black's law dictionary (5th ed.). (1979). St. Paul, MN: West Publishing Company.

Black's law dictionary (8th ed.). (2004). Retrieved from http://west.thomson.com/home

Black's law dictionary (9th abr. ed.). (2010, p. 240). St. Paul, MN: West Publishing Company.

Blatt, R., Brown, M., & Lerner, J. (n.d.). *Co-mediation: A success story at Chicago's Rush Medical Center.* Retrieved from http://www.adrsystems.com/news/co-mediation.pdf

Boulay, D. M., & Grant, P. D. (2011). Dispute resolution for nurses. In P. D. Grant & D. C. Ballard (Eds.), *Law for nurse leaders* (pp. 327–361). New York, NY: Springer Publishing Company.

Bovio, H. H. (2009). *Elder mediation matters: Probate, guardianship and family caregiving.* Retrieved from http://www.mediate.com/search.cfm

Brenner, H., & Bal, S. (2010). *Summary judgment in medical malpractice: The case of Hoard v. Roper Hospital.* Retrieved January 29, 2013, from www.healio.com/orthopedics/business-of-orthopedics/news/print/summaryjudgment-in-medical-malpractice-the-case-of hoard-v-roper-hospital

Brous, E. (2011). Patient rights and ethical considerations. In P. D. Grant & D. C. Ballard (Eds.), *Law for nurse leaders* (pp. 217–247). New York, NY: Springer Publishing Company.

Brous, E., Boulay, D. M., & Burger, V. (2011). The nurse and documentation. In P. D. Grant & D. C. Ballard (Eds.), *Law for nurse leaders* (pp. 175–189). New York, NY: Springer Publishing Company.

Burnham, G. M., & Rand, E. C. (2008). Disaster definitions. In *Public health guide for emergencies* (2nd ed., chap. 1). Baltimore, MD: Johns Hopkins Bloomberg School of Public Health. Retrieved from http://www.jhsph.edu/research/centers-and-institutes/center-for-refugee-and-disaster-response/publica tions_tools/publications/_CRDR_ICRC_Public_Health_Guide_ Book/Public_Health_Guide_for_Emergencies

Carter v. Norfolk Community Hospital Association, Inc., 761 F.2d 970 (4th Cir. 1985).

Centers for Disease Control and Prevention. (n.d.). *Public Health Emergency Law CDC foundational course for front-line practitioners version 3.1.* Retrieved from http://www.cdc.gov/phlp/docs/PHEL_ 3_1_unit_1_June_10_2009.pdf

Centers for Medicare & Medicaid Services. (n.d.) Retrieved from http://www.cms.hhs.gov/CFCsAndCOPs/

Centers for Medicare & Medicaid Services. (2006, July 13). *Memorandum Ref: S&C-06-21, "parking of emergency medical patient in hospital."* Baltimore, MD: Author.

Civil False Claims Act, 31 U.S.C. §§ 3729-33.

Civil Rights Act of 1866, 42 U.S.C. § 1981.

Civil Rights Act of 1871, 42 U.S.C. § 1983.

Coombes v. Florio, 450 Mass. 182 (2007).

Cruzan v. Harmon, 760 S.W.2d 408 (Mo. banc 1988).

Darling v. Charleston Hospital, 33 Ill.2d 236, 211 N.E.2d 253 (1965).

The District of Columbia Board of Nursing. (n.d.). *Discipline versus alternative program process.* Washington, DC: Author.

The District of Columbia Board of Nursing Committee on Impaired Nurses. (n.d.). Retrieved January 24, 2011, from http://doh .dc.gov/sites/default/files/dc/sites/doh/publication/attachments/ Nursing_Committee_on_Impaired_Nurses.pdf

Federal rules of evidence (F.R.E. 702). (2011). *Testimony by experts.* Retrieved January 28, 2013, from www.law.cornell.edu/rules/fre/ rule_702

Fisher & Phillips. (2006). *USERRA—The Uniformed Services Employment and Reemployment Rights Act*. Retrieved from http://www.laborlawyers.com/files/7741_USERRA%20Booklet%202006.pdf

Fisher, R., & Ury, W. (1981). *Getting to yes: Negotiating agreement without giving in*. Boston, MA: Houghton Mifflin.

42 C.F.R. § 482.13(g).

42 U.S.C. 5121 *et seq.*

42 U.S.C. 1320a-7b[b].

42 U.S.C. 1395nn.

Fowler, N. (1999). Corporate compliance: Framework and implementation. *Radiology Management, 21*(1), 50–53.

Grant, P. D. (1998). The nurse as an expert witness. In D. M. Rostant & R. F. Cady (Eds.), *AWHONN: Liability issues in perinatal nursing* (pp. 273–281). Philadelphia, PA: Lippincott.

Grant, P. D. (2011). The nurse and the law: A primer. In P. D. Grant & D. C. Ballard (Eds.), *Law for nurse leaders* (pp. 1–44). New York, NY: Springer Publishing Company.

Grant, P. D., & Reardon, N. J. (2011). Anatomy of civil and criminal trials. In P. D. Grant & D. C. Ballard (Eds.), *Law for nurse leaders* (pp. 300–326). New York, NY: Springer Publishing Company.

Grant, P. D., & Vecchione, J. J. (2011). Laws governing the workplace. In P. D. Grant & D. C. Ballard (Eds.), *Law for nurse leaders* (pp. 105–147). New York, NY: Springer Publishing Company.

Haney v. Alexander, 323 S.E.2d 430 (N.C. App. 1984).

Harris County Hospital District v. Joe Estrada et al., 872 S.W.2d 759 (1993).

Health Insurance Portability and Accountability Act of 1996, Pub. L No. 104-191.

Homeland Security Act of 2002, Pub. L. No. 107-296, 116 Stat. 2135 (2002), 6 U.S.C. §§ 101–557.

IPRO & Centers for Medicare and Medicaid Services. (2003). *Mediation dialogue*. Washington, DC: Author.

Karno, S. (2011). Nursing malpractice/negligence and liability. In P. D. Grant & D. C. Ballard (Eds.), *Law for nurse leaders* (pp. 249–280). New York, NY: Springer Publishing Company.

Kraus v. New Rochelle Hospital, 628 N.Y.S.2d 361 (N.Y. App. 1995).

Lama v. Borras, 16 F.3d 473 (1st Cir. 1994).

Liang, B. A. (2008). Government powers in emergencies and disasters: Permitted actions to protect the public's health. *Journal of Biolaw & Business, 11*(4), 37–41. Retrieved from http://anesthesia.ucsd.edu/research/faculty-research/Documents/LiangPubHealthJBB.pdf

McCarthy, F. X. (2007). *Federal Stafford Act disaster assistance: Presidential declarations, eligible activities, and funding* (CRS 7-5700). Washington, DC: Congressional Research Service.

Meritor Savings Bank v. Vinson, 47 U.S. 57 (1986).

Michael, J. (2003). What home healthcare nurses should know about fraud and abuse. *Home Healthcare Nurse, 21*(8), 522–530.

Miller, P. (2011). Risk management. In P. D. Grant & D. C. Ballard (Eds.), *Law for nurse leaders* (pp. 149–174). New York, NY: Springer Publishing Company.

Nathanson, M. J. (1993). Hospital corporate negligence: Enforcing the hospital's role of administrator. *Tort and Insurance Law Journal, 28*, 575–595.

National Institutes of Health. (2012). *Bioethics and the NIH*. Retrieved from http://bioethics.od.nih.gov/withinnih.html

Nieto v. Kappoor, 268 F.3d.1208 (10th Cir. 2001).

Noll, D. E. (2004). Bioethical mediation: Peacemaking and end of life conflicts. *Mediate.com Newsletter*. Retrieved from http://www.Mediate.com/articles/noll13cfm

Nursing licensure compact: Fact sheet for licensees and nursing students. (2010). Retrieved August 12, 2012, from www.ncsbn.org/SUD-10.pdf

Office of the Inspector General. (2008). *Annual performance report for fiscal year 2008*. Retrieved from http://oig.hhs.gov/publications/docs/budget/FY2008_APR.pdf

Patient Self Determination Act, Omnibus Reconciliation Act of 1990, Pub. L No. 101-158.

Pierce v. Ortho Pharmaceutical Corporation, 417 A.2d 505 (N.J. 1980).

Quinlan 70 N.J. 10, 355 A.2d 647 (NJ 1976)

Sarin v. Samaritan Health Care Center, 813 F.2d 755 (6th Cir. 1987).

Schiavo Ex. Rel Schindler v. Schiavo, 404 F.3d 1270 (11th Cir. 2005).

Seavers v. Methodist Medical Center of Oak Ridge, 9 S.W.3d 86 (Tenn. 1999).

Sermchief v. Gonzales, 660 S.W.2d 683 (Mo. banc 1983).

6 U.S.C. § 312(6).

Smith, R. K. (1999). *Corporate compliance in healthcare: A market-ing framework*. Retrieved from http://sbaer.uca.edu/Research/sma/1999/27.pdf

Standler, R. B. (2000). *Professional ethics and wrongful discharge* (pp. 1–24). Retrieved from http://www.Rbs2.com/ethics.htm

Sullivan v. Edward Hospital, et al., 806 N.E. 645 (Il. S.Ct. 2004).

Texas Nurses Association. (2012). *Winkler County nurses* (pp. 1–14). Retrieved from http://www.texasnurses.org/displaycommon.cfm?an=1subarticlenbr=509

Title VII of the Civil Rights Act of 1964, 42 U.S.C. § 2000 (e) *et seq.*

Toussaint v. Blue Cross, Blue Shield, 292 N.W.2d 880 (Mich. 1980).

Uniformed Services Employment and Reemployment Rights Act of 1994, Pub. L No. 103-353, 38 U.S.C. 4301-4334 (1994).

Unprofessional Conduct, 3 V.S.A. Section 129(a) 1-15, (b)1,2 (c).

Weinstock, D. S., & Chopko, C. M. (2008). Developing and sup-porting theories of hospital liability in catastrophic injury cases. *Feldman Shepherd Wohlgelernter Tanner Weinstock & Dodig.* Retrieved from http://www.feldmanshepherd.com

Weyandt v. Mason's Stores, Inc., 270 F. Supp. 283 (W.D. Pa. 1968).

Winkelman v. Beloit Memorial Hospital, 483 N.W.2d 211 (1992).

Wong v. Stripling, 881 F.2d 200 (5th Cir. 1989).

Additional Readings

Fowler, D. M. (Ed.). (2008). *Guide to the code of ethics for nurses: Interpretation and application*. College Park, MD: American Nurses Association.

Kjervik, D., & Brous, E. A. (2010). *Law and ethics for advanced prac-tice nursing.* New York, NY: Springer Publishing Company.

Index

Printed in the United States
By Bookmasters